SpringerBriefs in Public Health

SpringerBriefs in Child Health

Series Editor

Angelo P. Giardino, Department of Pediatrics
University of Utah
Salt Lake City, UT, USA

SpringerBriefs in Child Health present concise summaries of cutting-edge research and practical applications from the felds of child and adolescent health. This book series is designed to target children's health issues from birth through adolescence, from both a policy and practice perspective. Each subject in the series will be written by a specialist in that area. Their expertise will offer evaluation of the special health issues that would be of value to any health care provider. The authors all practice at nationally recognized children's hospitals and have done extensive research in their respective areas. The "template" for the series will be in three sections:

- "Snapshot from the Field" will address current practice and policy
- "Implications for Policy and Practice" will deal with the emerging science and best practices related to cutting edge work going on in the feld
- "Looking Ahead" will look forward towards anticipated changes, recommendations and strategies to achieve the best for children and families.

Featuring compact volumes of 55 to 125 pages, the series covers a range of content from professional to academic. Possible volumes in the series may consist of timely reports of state-of-the art analytical techniques, reports from the feld, snapshots of hot and/or emerging topics, elaborated theses, literature reviews, and in-depth case studies. Both solicited and unsolicited manuscripts are considered for publication in this series. Briefs are published as part of Springer's eBook collection, with millions of users worldwide. In addition, Briefs are available for individual print and electronic purchase. Briefs are characterized by fast, global electronic dissemination, standard publishing contracts, easy-to-use manuscript preparation and formatting guidelines, and expedited production schedules. We aim for publication 8-12 weeks after acceptance.

Claudia Delgado-Corcoran • Ryann Bierer
Lauren Cramer Finnerty • Katie Gradick
Brandy Harman • Mark Harousseau
Brooke Johnston • Sydney Kronaizl
Dominic Moore • Benjamin Moresco
Betsy Ostrander • Paige Patterson
Holly Spraker-Perlman • Amanda L. Thompson
Antonia Vitela-Elliott

Specialized Pediatric Palliative Care

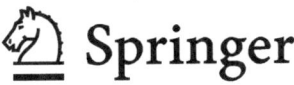 Springer

Claudia Delgado-Corcoran
Divisions of Critical Care and Palliative Care
Department of Pediatrics
University of Utah
Salt Lake City, UT, USA

Lauren Cramer Finnerty
Pediatric Advanced Care Team, Boston Children's
Hospital
Dana-Farber Cancer Institute
Boston, MA, USA

Brandy Harman
Office of the Chair, Department of Pediatrics
University of Utah
Salt Lake City, UT, USA

Brooke Johnston
Division of Palliative Care, Department of Pediatrics
University of Utah
Salt Lake City, UT, USA

Dominic Moore
Division of Palliative Care, Department of Pediatrics
University of Utah
Salt Lake City, UT, USA

Betsy Ostrander
Division of Neurology, Department of Pediatrics
University of Utah
Salt Lake City, UT, USA

Holly Spraker-Perlman
Divisions of Hematology/Oncology and Palliative Care
Department of Pediatrics
University of Utah
Salt Lake City, UT, USA

Antonia Vitela-Elliott
Palliative Care Services, Primary Children's Hospital
Intermountain Healthcare
Salt Lake City, UT, USA

Ryann Bierer
Divisions of Neonatology and Palliative Care
Department of Pediatrics
University of Utah
Salt Lake City, UT, USA

Katie Gradick
Division of Palliative Care, Department of Pediatrics
University of Utah
Salt Lake City, UT, USA

Mark Harousseau
Divisions of Palliative Care and Hospital Medicine
Department of Pediatrics
University of Utah
Salt Lake City, UT, USA

Sydney Kronaizl
Palliative Care Services, Primary Children's Hospital
Intermountain Healthcare
Salt Lake City, UT, USA

Benjamin Moresco
Division of Palliative Care, Department of Pediatrics
University of Utah
Salt Lake City, UT, USA

Paige Patterson
Departments of Pediatrics and Internal Medicine
University of Utah
Salt Lake City, UT, USA

Amanda L. Thompson
Pediatric Programs, Life with Cancer
Inova Schar Cancer Institute
Fairfax, VA, USA

ISSN 2192-3698   ISSN 2192-3701   (electronic)
SpringerBriefs in Public Health
ISSN 2625-2872   ISSN 2625-2880
SpringerBriefs in Child Health
ISBN 978-3-031-65451-0   ISBN 978-3-031-65452-7   (eBook)
https://doi.org/10.1007/978-3-031-65452-7

This Springer imprint is published by the registered company Springer Nature Switzerland AG
The registered company address is: Gewerbestrasse 11, 6330 Cham, Switzerland

If disposing of this product, please recycle the paper.

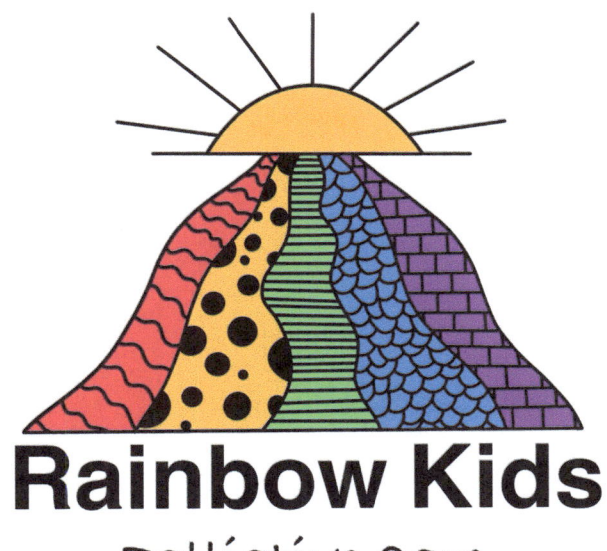

Rainbow Kids: A logo used by the palliative care service at author institution.
(Created by and used with permission from S. Josh Ware and Kari Yurth)

Foreword

Simply put, pediatric palliative care is increasingly recognized as an essential element in the comprehensive set of services and support that are necessary to care for children who are dealing with serious illness in a compassionate manner. The authors of this monograph provide us with a broad overview of the many details that define the "what" and "how" of state-of-the-art pediatric palliative care as we now understand it. Perhaps more importantly, these valued colleagues also give us a window into the "why" of pediatric palliative care, which we could describe as being our collective way to alleviate the suffering that the pediatric patient and their family experience as they navigate through an illness and care plan. The centrality of the connection between the work pediatric palliative care professionals do and the motivation that seems to routinely animate them is captured by the word "compassion." Drs. Trzeciak and Massarelli, in their now classic book entitled *Compassionomics: The Revolutionary Scientific Evidence That Caring Makes a Difference*, define compassion as "the emotional response to another's pain or suffering, involving an authentic desire to help" (2019, p. 5). One could make the case that it is exactly this "authentic desire to help" that defines the field of pediatric palliative care. Dr. Brené Brown's description of compassion characterizes well the pediatric palliative care occurring in our midst: "the daily practice of recognizing and accepting our shared humanity so that we treat ourselves and others with loving-kindness, and we take action in the face of suffering" (2021, p. 118). On an almost daily basis, those of us in pediatric health care actually witness the "authentic desire to help" combined with "action in the face of suffering" among our palliative care colleagues. Seeing their work in action assists those of us who are less skilled with how best to alleviate suffering and remain hopeful with the child and family with whom we are engaged in care.

As the authors of this monograph make clear, pediatric palliative care is a dynamic emerging sub-specialty within the broader area of pediatrics, and it is consummately an interdisciplinary effort that involves a number of professionals from a variety of other related fields. The definition of palliative care offered by the World Health Organization (WHO) (2020) best captures its comprehensive nature:

Palliative care is an approach that improves the quality of life of patients (adults and children) and their families who are facing problems associated with life-threatening illness. It prevents and relieves suffering through the early identification, correct assessment, and treatment of pain and other problems, whether physical, psychosocial, or spiritual. Addressing suffering involves taking care of issues beyond physical symptoms. Palliative care uses a team approach to support patients and their caregivers.

Each of these interdependent team members makes a unique and essential contribution to understanding the needs of a given child and their family and helps craft a care plan that optimizes what health care has to offer.

In addition to discussing the concepts of the palliative care approach referred to the WHO's definition, the authors point out a number of challenges confronting their emerging field of practice. There is well-documented variability in access to pediatric palliative care services, both nationally and internationally, with more availability present in the United States at academic settings, most notably in the nation's children's hospitals and health systems. Not uncommonly, palliative care is not well understood by the lay public nor by providers in the healthcare field and is still confused with hospice care. While palliative care can include hospice services delivered to patients near end of life, it is much broader and not limited to end-of-life care.

Additionally, the authors provide us with information about specific populations of children that are likely to be served by pediatric palliative care teams, including those children seen in oncology, cardiology, and neurology as well as those with a variety of chronic and/or disabling conditions. The authors also offer valuable insights into the venues of care, spanning inpatient, outpatient, and home care settings. The data on the growth of pediatric palliative care teams is encouraging, but the obvious mismatch between the need for pediatric palliative care and the number of pediatric palliative care sub-specialists available to serve is striking. The authors issue a realistic call to action to close the gap between those who need pediatric palliative care and the number of skilled professionals necessary to provide that care in the coming decades. This call to action revolves around broader recognition of the importance of education and training in pediatric palliative care, continued prioritization of research and evaluation in order to expand the evidence base for such care, and increased attention to ongoing sustainable funding to support the delivery of this care to all children and families in need.

Reading through the material in this monograph, the essential nature of pediatric palliative care in the alleviation of suffering among seriously affected children and their families is clear. The connection between palliative care and the authentic desire to help is palpable and defines compassion. Whether in the field of pediatric palliative care itself or as one among the many who benefit from the work of pediatric palliative care providers, our collective responsibility remains to encourage and support those who courageously come forward to serve in this compassionate manner. The ensuing pages make the imperative clear: pediatric palliative care is the healthcare system's way of showing children and their families that we care about helping them as they navigate through the many twists and turns along their healthcare journey. Let's all commit to doing our part to help alleviate suffering by advocating for and taking steps toward greater pediatric palliative care capability and availability in our healthcare settings for all children and families who may be in need.

Angelo P. Giardino
W.T. Gibson Presidential Professor and Chair
Department of Pediatrics
University of Utah School of Medicine
Salt Lake City, UT, USA

Chief Medical Officer, Intermountain Primary
Children's Hospital
Salt Lake City, UT, USA

March 2024

References

Brown, B. (2021). *Atlas of the heart: Mapping meaningful connection and the language of human experience*. Random House.

Trzciek, S., & Mazzarelli, A. (2019). *Compassionomics: The revolutionary scientific evidence that caring makes a difference.* Studer Group.

World Health Organization. (2020, August 5). *Palliative care*. Retrieved March 27, 2024, from https://www.who.int/news-room/fact-sheets/detail/palliative-care

Acknowledgments

The authors would like to thank Katie Boner, MA, BCC, Former Palliative Care Chaplain; Stacey Bushell, CPNP, Palliative Care Nurse Practitioner; Jessaca Condas, BSN, RN, Palliative Care Nurse/Care Coordinator; Anne Harvey, DNP, BCC, Palliative Care Nurse Practitioner; Kelly Kelso, CPNP, Palliative Care Nurse Practitioner; Allie Kendall, DNP, NNP-BC, Palliative Care Nurse Practitioner; Brittney Moss, LCSW, Palliative Care Social Worker; Sharon Noorda, BSN, RN, Palliative Care Nurse/Care Coordinator; Ashley Peter, LCSW, Palliative Care Manager; Jamie Seale, NNP-BC, Palliative Care Nurse Practitioner; Tomoko Tsukamoto, MSN, RN, Palliative Care Nurse/Care Coordinator; and Kari Yurth, CMHC, Mental Health Therapist, for their expertise, support, and assistance in preparing the manuscript and for being part of a great team.

Contents

About the Authors

Claudia Delgado-Corcoran, MD, MPH is an Associate Professor of Pediatrics at the University of Utah and works in the Divisions of Pediatric Critical Care Medicine and Palliative Care at Primary Children's Hospital in Salt Lake City, Utah. She is originally from Colombia, South America and has lived in the United States since the early 1990s. She did her medical school studies in Colombia and earned a Master of Public Health (MPH) degree from the University of South Carolina. She completed Pediatric Residency and Pediatric Critical Care Medicine fellowship at the University of Florida and completed a year-long training in Cardiac Intensive Care at Arkansas Children's Hospital. She joined the University of Utah in 2009, and since that time she has been working in the Cardiac Intensive Care Unit (CICU) at Primary Children's Hospital in Salt Lake City. Additionally, she completed a fellowship in hospice and palliative care medicine in June 2020 at the University of Utah. She is board-certified in Pediatrics, Pediatric Critical Care Medicine, and Palliative Care and Hospice Medicine. She has almost 20 years of clinical work experience in Critical Care. Her research work in the last few years has focused on increasing the involvement of palliative care in children with serious illness, particularly children with heart disease. She also champions grieving sessions after the death of every child in the Pediatric and Cardiac ICUs at Primary Children's Hospital. Her hobbies include traveling with her husband and two kids, and dancing, particularly to music from her native country.

Ryann Bierer, MD is an Assistant Professor in Neonatology and Pediatric Palliative Care at the University of Utah and Primary Children's Hospital. She provides neonatology services at three facilities: the neonatal intensive care units (NICUs) at University of Utah Hospital, Primary Children's Hospital, and Intermountain Medical Center. She also completed a fellowship in Hospice and Palliative Medicine at the University of Utah in 2018 and now provides pediatric palliative care with the Rainbow Kids Palliative Care team at Primary Children's Hospital.

Lauren Cramer Finnerty, MSW, LICSW   is a clinical social worker specializing in pediatric palliative care with the Pediatric Advanced Care Team (PACT) at Boston Children's Hospital and the Dana Farber Cancer Institute. Lauren has recently begun developing her new role as the dedicated ambulatory pediatric palliative care social worker for PACT. She completed the Harvard Interprofessional Palliative Care Fellowship after earning her Master of Social Work with a Certificate of Graduate Studies in Childhood and Adolescent Trauma from Rhode Island College. Lauren holds undergraduate degrees in Social Work and Psychology from Providence College. In addition to her palliative care work, Lauren provides individual and family cognitive behavioral therapy to children, adolescents, and young adults with anxiety disorders in Massachusetts.

Katie Gradick, MD, MHS   received her undergraduate degree in Applied Social Ethics from Harvard College, her medical degree from the University of Wisconsin School of Medicine and Public Health, and Master of Health Science from the Johns Hopkins Bloomberg School of Medicine and Public Health in Baltimore, Maryland. She completed her internship at the Massachusetts General Hospital for Children and her Pediatrics residency and Hospice and Palliative Medicine fellowship at the University of Utah.

Dr. Gradick's clinical interests include trainee wellness, language inclusivity, and anti-racist health care reform. She is a member of the American Academy of Pediatrics, American Academy of Hospice and Palliative Medicine, and the Gold Humanism Honor Society. She also serves as the University of Utah Site Director for the Global Hospice and Palliative Medicine Fellowship in collaboration with St. Jude's Children's Research Hospital and the Unidad Nacional de Oncología Pediátrica in Guatemala. Dr. Gradick is an Assistant Professor at the University of Utah in the Division of Pediatric Palliative Care.

Brandy Harman, BA   has worked in the Department of Pediatrics at the University of Utah since 2010. She is an administrator in the Office of the Department Chair and spends much of her time coaching faculty on writing skills and editing their manuscripts. She enjoys helping fellow team members express their ideas and research results clearly and succinctly and finds great delight in coming across a well-written phrase. With several years of exposure to myriad topics in the field of pediatric medicine, she has a little knowledge about a lot of areas and appreciates any opportunity to add to her understanding. She is particularly interested in equitable access and treatment in health care as well as mental health services and support for professional and family caregivers.

Mark Harousseau, MD   received his medical degree from New York Medical College. He then completed residency in Pediatrics at the University of Utah and served a fourth year as chief resident. He completed his fellowship in Hospice and Palliative Medicine in the pediatric track at the University of Utah and has continued on as faculty with clinical responsibilities in the Division of Pediatric Palliative Care on the Rainbow Kids Palliative Care team and in the Division of Pediatric

Hospital Medicine. His clinical interests include palliative education in pediatric residency, pediatric hospice care, and effective communication around serious illness.

Brooke Johnston, MD   graduated from Morehouse School of Medicine in Atlanta, Georgia. She completed residency in Pediatrics at the University of Utah, remaining for an additional year of chief residency. Dr. Johnston was a fellow in Pediatric Hospice and Palliative Medicine at Akron Children's Hospital in Akron, Ohio. Following training, she worked in inpatient and in-home pediatric hospice and palliative care in the University of South Carolina Upstate.

Dr. Johnston is an Assistant Professor of Pediatrics and serves as a Faculty House Mentor for medical students at the Spencer Fox Eccles School of Medicine at the University of Utah. Her interests include medical communication, behavioral health components of medical experiences, and community-based efforts to address social determinants of health.

Sydney Kronaizl, MS, CCLS   is a Certified Child Life Specialist in the Neonatal Intensive Care Unit at Primary Children's Hospital where she provides patient and family support for critically ill infants. She has also worked as a Clinical Research Coordinator for Rainbow Kids Palliative Care. Her research interests include children's understanding of death and developmentally appropriate support. When she is not working, Sydney enjoys traveling, cooking, and spending time with her partner and pup.

Dominic Moore, MD   is the Senior Medical Director of Hospice and Palliative Care for Intermountain Healthcare Canyons Region, where his mission is to ensure the highest quality care is available to all people with serious illness. Dr. Moore also serves as the Division Chief for Pediatric Palliative Care and Associate Program Director for the Hospice and Palliative Medicine Fellowship. He is a member of the Gold Humanism Honor Society and has focused his academic work on responsible prescribing, self-care for providers, and the role that spirituality plays in healthcare interactions. He is focused on improving the health and life experience of communities through outreach to encourage advance care planning and has worked with partners throughout the intermountain region to accomplish this.

Benjamin Moresco, MD   is originally from Idaho and currently serves as the medical director on the Rainbow Kids Palliative Care team at Primary Children's Hospital as a pediatrician and palliative care specialist. He received his medical degree from the University of Washington School of Medicine as part of the WWAMI program—a multi-state medical education program serving Washington, Wyoming, Alaska, Montana, and Idaho. He completed his Pediatric residency followed by chief residency at the Children's Hospital of San Antonio/Baylor College of Medicine as part of the first residency class in San Antonio, Texas. He then completed his fellowship in Pediatric Hospice and Palliative Care in Boston, Massachusetts, at the Harvard Interprofessional Fellowship Program working clinically with children cared for at Brigham and Women's Hospital, Dana Farber Cancer Institute, and Boston Children's Hospital.

Dr. Moresco's clinical interests include comprehensive care for children with special healthcare needs, bereavement, telehealth, rural medicine, and complex pain/symptom management for children with serious illness. When not at work, he enjoys spending time with his superstar wife (who you may know, Gabby Robuccio), and dogs. He also does many of the stereotypical Utah activities like hiking, biking, fishing, and skiing.

Betsy Ostrander, MD is an Associate Professor of Pediatric Neurology at the University of Utah. She attended Loyola Strich School of Medicine and completed her pediatric residency at RUSH Children's Hospital. She is the Director of the Fetal and Neonatal Neurology Program. Her clinical focus is infants with neurological disorders and those at high risk for neurodevelopmental impairments. She also is the Director of the NeuroICU consult service, providing neurology consultation for critically ill children. She leads the Early Diagnosis for Cerebral Palsy effort implemented in 2018 and has taught the neurological exam and early cerebral palsy implementation tools in the United States and several other countries.

Paige Patterson, MD is an internal medicine/pediatric physician with specialty training in hospice and palliative medicine. She is an Assistant Professor at the University of Utah in the Internal Medicine and Pediatrics departments. She serves as the Medical Director for two pediatric-focused hospices in the Salt Lake valley, as well as serving on the Utah Compassionate Use Board to approve compassionate use of medical cannabis for patients under the age of 21. She is co-director of a transition to medical school course, as well as the Utah Certificate of Palliative Education course offered twice yearly to members of the healthcare community. She practices mostly outpatient palliative care and is dedicated to improving home-based palliative care for patients in the area.

Holly Spraker-Perlman, MD, MS, FAAHPM, ABOIM is an Associate Professor in the Department of Pediatrics, Divisions of Pediatric Palliative Care and Pediatric Hematology-Oncology at the University of Utah/Primary Children's Hospital. She received her undergraduate degree at the College of William and Mary in Williamsburg, Virginia (BS Biology), and then received her Medical Doctor degree (MD) from Virginia Commonwealth University in Richmond, Virginia. She completed a Pediatrics residency at Emory University in Atlanta, Georgia. Her fellowship training for both Pediatric Hematology-Oncology and Hospice and Palliative Medicine were completed at St. Jude Children's Research Hospital in Memphis, TN. Dr. Spraker-Perlman worked in the Division of Pediatric Hematology-Oncology at the University of Utah/Primary Children's Hospital from 2010 through 2017 and transitioned back to St. Jude Children's Research Hospital as a clinician researcher on the Palliative Oncology Team at St. Jude Children's Research Hospital from 2017 to 2023. She then returned to the University of Utah as a faculty member of the Rainbow Kids Palliative Care team as well as in the Division of Pediatric

Hematology-Oncology, focused on pediatric solid tumors. Dr. Spraker-Perlman is also board certified in Integrative Medicine and trained in pediatric massage and acupuncture. Dr. Spraker-Perlman's research interests include honest prognostic communication in the field of pediatric oncology and complementary and integrative symptom management for children undergoing cancer therapy. She enjoys reading, hiking, crafting, and spending time with her husband, son, and dogs.

Amanda L. Thompson, PhD   currently serves as Chief of Pediatric Psychology and Director of Pediatric Programs at Life with Cancer, the psychosocial program of the Inova Schar Cancer Institute in Fairfax, VA. Dr. Thompson completed her PhD in Clinical-Developmental Psychology at the University of Pittsburgh, her predoctoral residency at Nemours Children's Hospital in Wilmington, DE, and her post-doctoral fellowship at Nationwide Children's Hospital in Columbus, Ohio.

Dr. Thompson has a national presence as an author of the Standards of Psychosocial Care for Children with Cancer and their Families and as project lead for the development of Competencies for Psychologists in Pediatric Palliative Care. She currently serves as Co-chair of the American Psychosocial Oncology Society's Pediatrics/AYA Special Interest Group, APA's representative to the Pediatrics Division of the National Coalition of Hospice and Palliative Medicine, and a board member on the Pediatrics Council of the American Academy of Hospice and Palliative Medicine. Her interests include pediatric psycho-oncology, palliative and end-of-life care, grief and loss, program development, interdisciplinary team collaboration, and mentorship. When not at work, Dr. Thompson feeds her infinite wanderlust by traveling any- and everywhere and capturing it all through her favorite hobby of photography.

Antonia Vitela-Elliott, PhD, CCLS   is a certified child life specialist on the pediatric palliative care team at Primary Children's Hospital in Salt Lake City, Utah. She specializes in providing bereavement support to patients and their families, as well as normalizing the hospital environment so that no matter the prognosis, a child or teen has opportunities to feel normal. Her research interests are in legacy building and patient advocacy.

Chapter 1
Introduction and Definitions

1.1 Introduction to Palliative Care

This volume of *SpringerBriefs in Child Health* will introduce you to the field and practice of pediatric palliative care (PPC). It is written by colleagues devoted to the care of children with serious illness, and we hope that it will help you care for these special patients and their families.

Palliative care as a term was first used by Dr. Balfour Mount in 1974 to describe holistic caring for the seriously ill. It has evolved into a multidisciplinary medical specialty with fellowship training, board certification, and acceptance as a standard of serious illness care (Clark, 2007). This field is focused on providing value-concordant care for the body, mind, and spirit of a patient and those who care for them, including their health care team. The term was chosen based on the Latin word *palliare*, meaning "to cloak." This original meaning echoes in the description of palliative care as an "extra layer of support."

Long before the term "palliative" was coined, an old tradition of caring for the dying was restored and renewed in Western medicine by Dame Cecily Saunders, MD—now recognized as the first leader of the hospice movement (Clark, 2007). The field that grew initially from these roots continues to be inclusive of hospice care but has expanded to care for patients at the time of—and occasionally in the process of—diagnosis. Some PPC patients benefit from service during the fetal and perinatal period thanks to advances in technology and practice that can help expectant parents prepare for all possible outcomes in their children (Rossfeld et al., 2019).

Although many of the early leaders in palliative care had a sense of the pediatric implications of this field, the roots of palliative care are in adult medicine and have since expanded into pediatric care. Early pediatric leaders in the field are still clinically active and influencing subsequent generations. The first PPC services grew out of departments or divisions with vision and budget to allow for development and experimentation in the field. Pediatric oncology, anesthesia, and hospital medicine were frequently the home of this developing specialty, with a wide variety of additional homes as the field has expanded (Sisk et al., 2020). In 2024, pediatric palliative care has become an increasingly independent presence in pediatric departments, with a record number of dedicated divisions.

Both a historical and contemporary lens in pediatric health is useful in considering the emergence, work, and future of pediatric palliative care. While mortality risk is decreasing and average lifespan is increasing, there is still a significant group of people who never make it to adulthood or have a significantly compromised survival based on the diagnosis that they carry. Some of these children do not live past delivery or even infancy, but a growing number are living beyond historical expectations thanks to advancements in pediatric medicine (Sisk et al., 2020). Interestingly, the same advances that make prolonged life an option have also extended the window of time in which a fatal or threatening diagnosis can be known. The new frontiers of fetal medicine, including fetal surgery, have given families and care teams knowledge of problems that are likely to be serious or even fatal from a much earlier age—sometimes months before an expected delivery (American Academy of Pediatrics [AAP], 2019). The new group of surviving children and young adults is often facing extended, though still limited, prospects. The life of a seriously ill patient has much improved in the past century, and a portion of that improvement is thanks to pediatric palliative care. Patients can endure treatments and life-prolonging measures in better comfort and health than ever before as teams work to care for the whole patient.

Modern pediatric medicine benefits from the work of palliative care as providers endeavor "to cure sometimes, to relieve often, and to comfort always" (Kumar & Allaudeen, 2016). We hope that as you review this volume of *SpringerBriefs in Child Health*, you will better understand how you and your patients can benefit from this young but quickly maturing field.

1.2 Definition of Terms Commonly Used in Palliative and Hospice Care

Pediatric Palliative Care

Palliative care for children expands the concept of total care of a patient's physical, emotional, social, and spiritual well-being, and applies it to enhancing the quality of life of children and families as they navigate life-threatening conditions and associated suffering.

Pediatric Hospice

Hospice provides compassionate care for a child with a terminal diagnosis and life expectancy of less than 6 months. Hospice care supports families through a care plan developed by an interdisciplinary team of experts that focuses on spiritual and emotional support, as well as medical care, including symptom management.

Quality of Life

A central concept to palliative care, quality of life is an individual's own definition of meaningful measures of physical, psychological, emotional, and spiritual health. Quality-of-life goals are often considered in the context of medical decisions.

Illness Trajectories

In pediatric palliative care, there are usually four illness pathways that contribute to a child's illness and possible death:

1. A potentially curable illness where treatment fails
2. An expected premature death despite disease-modifying treatments
3. A progressive condition with no curative treatment available
4. A non-progressive condition with associated high morbidity leading to early death

Anticipatory Grief

The physical, emotional, and spiritual response to an anticipated loss. Often more pronounced in younger patients with no prior exposure to grief and loss. Anticipatory grief is often associated with unrecognized intense emotions.

Baseline

A term used to identify a period of stability in a child's condition where features of the illness (extent of disease, response to treatment, dependency on medical technology, functional status) are not changing significantly. Baselines and "new baselines" are at times unclear and more subjective. Clear deterioration from a baseline can signal a changing illness trajectory (see above).

Shared Decision-Making

An approach to developing a care plan for a child that considers medical recommendations as they relate to a family's goals and expertise in navigating their child's illness.

Life-Sustaining Therapies

Therapies that are used to prolong life with artificial means. This includes mechanical ventilation, enteric and parental feeding, dialysis and continuous renal replacement therapy (CRRT), and extracorporeal membrane oxygenation (ECMO). It can also include therapies such as oxygen supplementation, bilevel positive airway pressure (BIPAP), continuous positive airway pressure (CPAP), intravenous hydration, antibiotics, and certain other medications (e.g., inotropes and pressors). Devices such as implanted defibrillators, pacemakers, and ventricular assistive devices may also be considered life-sustaining therapies.

Total Pain

There are many different types of pain. Nociceptive pain is pain related to tissue injury and inflammation from noxious or impending damage to structures in the body. Neuropathic pain is pain that results from injury to the sensory nervous system (which can be peripheral or central). Total pain is pain that encompasses all the aspects of a person's physical, psychological, social, spiritual, and practical struggles. Varying pain sources compound and muddle the experience of pain. For example, a teenager may have physical pain from bony metastatic lesions, distress about missing summer camp, and worry about how their family feels. This may compound the experience of physical pain. Considering all the dimensions of total pain is vital to appropriate palliative care of seriously ill patients and to adequately treating pain and suffering.

Opioids

Natural, synthetic, or semisynthetic chemicals that interact with opioid receptors on nerve cells in the body and brain and reduce the intensity of pain signals and feelings of pain. This class of drugs includes the illegal drug heroin, synthetic opioids such as fentanyl, and opiate-based pain medications available legally by prescription, such as oxycodone, hydrocodone, codeine, morphine, and many others. Prescription opioids are generally safe when taken for a short time and as directed by a doctor, but because they produce euphoria in addition to pain relief, they can be misused and have addiction potential.

Although the terms "opiates" and "opioids" are often used interchangeably, they are different: opiates refer to natural opioids such as heroin, morphine, and codeine; opioids refer to all natural, semisynthetic, and synthetic opioids.

Delirium

Delirium is an acute, fluctuating alteration of mental status, evidenced by waxing and waning deficits in attention, cognition, and consciousness. It is usually reversible, unless it is terminal delirium (see below). There are several clinical tools available to assess delirium in various settings and at various developmental stages. Delirium is more common in older adults and is likely underrecognized in young non- or not-yet verbal patients. Delirium can be divided into subtypes: hypoactive delirium, hyperactive delirium, and mixed. Hypoactive delirium is often difficult to diagnose due to the subtle nature of its symptoms, which can be mistaken for symptoms of critical illness. Hyperactive delirium is often recognized because of the agitation patients experience; physical and psychiatric agitation often grabs clinicians' attention quickly.

Terminal delirium is delirium specific to the end of life. It is often hypoactive delirium; however, occasionally hyperactive delirium with severe agitation occurs and can be very distressing for families.

Certification of Terminal Illness

This is a statement signed by the patient's hospice physician that qualifies the patient for hospice. The statement must be signed within 2 days of admission to hospice and includes the hospice admitting diagnosis, comorbid conditions related to the terminal diagnosis, and a statement that the life expectancy is 6 months or less if the disease runs its natural course.

Orders for Life-Sustaining Therapies

These orders are known by varying names in different states, such as Provider Orders for Life-Sustaining Treatment, Medical Orders for Scope of Treatment, Physician Orders for Scope of Treatment, or Medical Orders for Life-Sustaining Treatment. These are legal, medical orders by a provider (i.e., physician, nurse practitioner, or physician assistant) that allow patients and families to specify what type and for how long life-sustaining therapies are acceptable for themselves and their loved ones. Legal requirements for the form, as well as the forms themselves, vary from state to state. Most typically address a few topics: Do Not Resuscitate (DNR) order, tube feeding/artificial hydration, intubation and mechanical ventilation, intensive care unit (ICU) level of care, and IV antibiotics or other treatment modalities that are sometimes foregone in end-of-life situations.

DNR
Do Not Resuscitate, also known as DNAR or Do Not Attempt to Resuscitate. If a patient or family selects this option and a patient's heart has stopped beating and/or they have stopped breathing, cardiopulmonary resuscitation (CPR) will not be initiated, and the patient will be allowed to die without medical intervention.

AND
Allow Natural Death. The course of treatment is identical to DNR, but phrasing emphasizes what will be done for the person receiving care, including aggressive symptom management as part of a holistic plan of care.

DNI
Do Not Intubate. This order may require additional stipulations, such as "Okay for BiPAP," as children often suffer respiratory failure before cardiovascular failure.

Bereavement
Bereavement is the experience when someone (or something) important to us is gone. While grief can continue indefinitely, bereavement in palliative care specifically refers to the immediate post-loss period. In the pediatric hospice setting, bereavement services are offered to family members of a child who has died—not just the parents, but also siblings, other important caregivers, and close family members. These services are usually provided by a social worker and/or a chaplain, and often continue officially for a year after the patient's death. Bereavement groups are often offered to those who have suffered an acute loss (i.e., patient was not seriously ill in hospice) as well. There are often parent and child-centered grief or bereavement groups, which may include resources such as art and music therapy.

1.3 Primary and Specialized Palliative Care

Primary palliative care refers to those aspects of palliative care provided by a primary care provider or team (Moresco & Moore, 2021; Rothschild & Derrington, 2020; Blume et al., 2023). The provision of such care is founded on the competence and comfort of team members regarding basic palliative care skills, including pain and symptom management; high-quality communication regarding prognosis, treatment, and goals of care; and care coordination to promote quality of life as it is defined by patients and their families (Moresco & Moore, 2021; Rothschild & Derrington, 2020; Blume et al., 2023). These competencies comprise a skillset necessary for every provider of care (Moresco & Moore, 2021) and can be gained in a variety of formats including fellowship, online resources, and workshop-based training (Rothschild & Derrington, 2020).

Specialty palliative care refers to those aspects of palliative care provided by a sub-specialty-trained palliative care team that possesses a larger depth and breadth of knowledge pertaining to palliative care. Skills specific to this level of care include complex or intensive symptom management, crucial communication, advance care planning, and provision of care, support, and resources at the end of life and in bereavement (Moresco & Moore, 2021; Rothschild & Derrington, 2020; Blume et al., 2023).

Primary and specialty palliative care are not mutually exclusive. Rather, specialty palliative care constitutes a complementary layer of support that can be provided in addition to primary palliative care when indicated (Moresco & Moore, 2021; Rothschild & Derrington, 2020; Blume et al., 2023). The current specialty pediatric palliative care workforce is unable to meet the needs of all children who would benefit from their services; the standard provision of primary palliative care bridges this gap as it allows team members to provide a basic level of palliative care and consult the subspecialty team as indicated (Moresco & Moore, 2021; Rothschild & Derrington, 2020). In short, the provision of primary palliative care ensures that those patients and families requiring such care maintain access to it, while simultaneously reserving the workforce of subspecialty-trained providers to meet the most complex and distressing needs (Moresco & Moore, 2021).

1.4 Clinical Areas of Focus in Palliative Care

In this section, we describe palliative care based on the functions of a team caring for patients with serious illness. Most palliative care teams have an interdisciplinary approach in which team members work collaboratively toward a shared care plan; this contrasts with the multidisciplinary approach of colleagues with distinct primary professional identities working in parallel. As would be expected, there is not a one-size-fits-all approach that every patient who sees a palliative care team will work through. Instead, this is a practical list of tools that is selected based on the given situation and how a patient and family will be best served. We will concentrate on medical communication, goal setting, advance care planning, symptom management, and connection along the care continuum (AAP, 2019). Many families who are served by palliative care have developed expertise in some of these areas. All families served by palliative care are treated as partners in this work (Schuetze et al., 2022).

1.4.1 Medical Communication

Palliative care teams focus on medical communication to ensure the most patient- and family-centered care possible. Shared decision-making starts with trust and shared understanding (Boland et al., 2019). In building a foundation of trust and communication, teams can assess medical literacy, past communication patterns, misunderstandings, language preference, and communication styles. Medical communication is a common reason for specialist palliative care consultation, with primary teams worrying that a patient or family "doesn't get it." Exploring this statement of concern often allows the multilayered considerations of a situation to be addressed. While occasionally it is truly an issue of a patient or family not being able to understand, more often it is a combined mismatch of medical literacy, preferred language, or communication style that leads to this perception (Katz et al., 2021). This is a two-way street as occasionally families feel they are being as clear as possible with a team, and yet their intent is misunderstood. In an early discussion, a palliative care team will elicit understanding with open-ended questions such as "what have your doctors told you about what is going on?" or "how do things seem to be going right now?" These questions are phrased in such a way as to allow a family to answer candidly without feeling there is a right or wrong answer. As discussed later in this edition, lack of a shared language can feel like a stumbling block for communicating with families. Palliative care teams play a critical role in advocating for and utilizing interpretive services with all families where appropriate (Delgado-Corcoran et al., 2022).

1.4.2   Goal Setting

Goals set by children and families facing serious illness are as diverse as the families themselves. Eliciting goals may be as simple as asking what people are hoping for. As an illness progresses, the questioning might be even more specific (e.g., "If you knew that time was short and measured in months, what would be the most important things to do?"). Even when there is a clear goal in mind, it can be difficult to share without prompting. Goals may range from the personal ("I want to make sure that I can go to school without tubes") to more community-focused ("I would like to be sure that my tumor is donated for research after my death"). Although rare early in a serious illness journey, it is not uncommon for goals to contradict each other as a disease progresses. Staying out of the hospital may begin to contradict the hope of taking advantage of every therapy, no matter how unique. Sometimes goals have an anchor that will not hold, such as a patient with a prognosis of months to a few years looking at plans that are decades away. In these cases, palliative care teams work with patients, families, and the primary team to find new anchors for hope and planning. This works to preserve hope while also helping with the acknowledgment of the important factors in a case (Kaye et al., 2023).

1.4.3   Advance Care Planning

Advance care planning is a blanket term for a wide range of considerations, conversations, and documentation that ensure a patient or family understands the potential serious situations they may find themselves in and provide an opportunity to explore decisions about their treatment before a crisis arises. These decisions and conversations often weigh heavily on patients and families, and yet these topics of conversation are often avoided. Normalizing the process in terms of "having an emergency plan" has significant power in diffusing concerns from patients and families. In most cases, patients under 18 years of age are required to have a parent involved and lead these conversations. Until adulthood, parents will sign legal documents related to advance care planning on the patient's behalf. However, as children grow and mature, they often have opinions and concerns of their own about the way they are treated in an emergency. Eliciting the patient's preferences for involvement in advance care planning will allow them to feel respected and involved as much as they might like to be. Many parents worry that involving children in these conversations will have a stressful effect. While it is important to follow a parent's lead, helping them see the benefits of transparency and empowerment of their child is part of the palliative role. Advance care planning in the pediatric population may also include helping parents prepare to advocate for their children into adulthood through guardianship and other mechanisms when appropriate. Specialist palliative care teams should have expertise and resources to aid in these and other discussions (Harmoney et al., 2019).

1.4.4   Symptom Management

Palliative care teams are specially designed to identify, address, and alleviate patient suffering. Symptom management is often multifactorial, and palliative care teams follow a biopsychosocial model in evaluating the needs of a patient (AAP, 2019). The physical aspects of suffering are the factors most commonly described in the literature, albeit that description still leaves much unknown. Specialists in palliative medicine can assess current and possible therapies to address suffering, which may come in many forms and are often underappreciated. These therapies are a mixture of pharmacologic and nonpharmacologic interventions that are selected with care to ensure the maximum benefit and minimum side effect when employed. Many of the medications used for severe or especially intense symptoms are uncommon in the pediatric world, leading to a lack of comfort by some in treating the symptoms of patients with serious illness. Palliative care collaborates with pharmacists and the primary team to find the best method of caring for the patient, even if that treatment is as unusual as continuous infusions. Later in this publication you will read more about the members of the palliative care team with expertise in psychosocial and spiritual support who complement the medical providers as they collaborate to treat the whole person. Social work and chaplaincy have long been part of the accepted standard interdisciplinary team, and they are increasingly joined by child life specialists, expressive therapists, and mental health professionals to further enhance symptom management.

1.4.5 Connection Along the Care Continuum

Palliative care in adults is often involved at the very end of a serious illness journey. While this happens in children, especially those on an aggressive treatment course, it is much more common that pediatric palliative care teams are called early in a disease process and interact multiple times with the patient and family (Lee et al., 2023). The team sees the patient and family as they transition between care settings, through the ups and downs of disease progression, and into the final stages of their disease (Fig. 1.1). These transitions present myriad opportunities for details, preferences, and histories to be mistaken, dropped, or forgotten. Problems within these transitions can be life threatening and shorten an already brief life. Palliative care teams should work as part of the overall care coordination process to ensure that patients are connected to care managers in their primary care provider or primary specialist office. They may also work closely with complex care teams, who have a unique role and often share patients with palliative care teams (Harris et al., 2023). A few programs have been created to address the unique problems of pediatric patients including the concurrent care hospice benefit (discussed later), Medicaid waivers that allow for consideration of medical need and complexity rather than income, and specialized practices for transitioning to adult care or addressing complex, chronic needs.

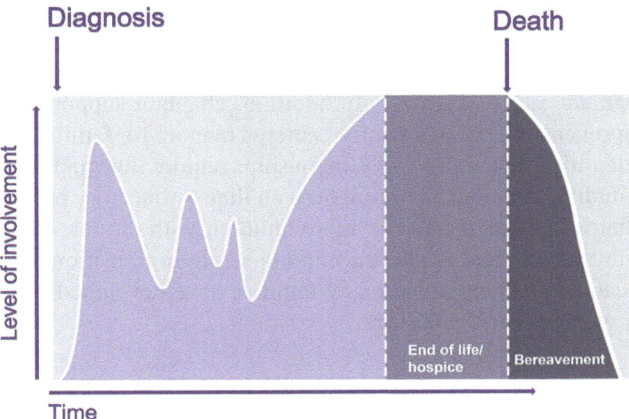

Fig. 1.1 Palliative care involvement in terminal illness

1.5   Unique Aspects of Pediatric Palliative Care

There are several distinctions of pediatric palliative care (PPC) that are worth considering. The complexities of chronic life-threatening pediatric illnesses lead to important decision-making dynamics within family units. PPC often involves decisions for a vulnerable population of patients and surrogate decision-makers. By virtue of chronological age, developmental age, and neurobehavioral baseline, clinicians in PPC are often exposed to the subtle balance between evolving autonomy and decision-making capacity in their patients. Furthermore, PPC is associated with significant uncertainty around prognosis, expanded interdisciplinary roles, and longer durations of specialized palliative services coinciding with disease-modifying and curative treatments. Families become integral caregivers and experts in the care of their child. Often learning advanced skills in medical technologies and clinical assessments, parents are active participants in providing care to a degree that is not necessarily common in adults. Furthermore, parents are responsible for informed consent, yet a child's autonomy and assent are normally balanced in the context of behavior and cognitive developments, which vary widely. A child's involvement in decision-making will also change with time and maturity. These nuances require significant time and expertise to navigate.

Pediatrics is susceptible to considerable uncertainty around prognosis. Trajectories, even in the most severe diagnoses, such as a fatal genetic condition, are often unpredictable, especially around end-of-life timing. Prognosis is influenced by important decisions regarding short- and long-term life-sustaining interventions. These implications open the possibility for extended stays in hospitals or admission to long-term care facilities. Dependency on medical technologies becomes an important factor that parents consider based on goals. These decisions must be weighed by families and their providers as they navigate severe illness in the face of significant uncertainty. PPC providers are an important source of support as these decisions are being made.

Lastly, with its expansive developmental scope, additional interdisciplinary team members are crucial to pediatric palliative care teams. This may include pediatric behavioral specialists and child life specialists, who have specialized training in child development and psychology. In addition, chaplain support can be vital to offering comprehensive care in a family-centered manner for families with religious or spiritual identities. Many of these relationships require time and frequent follow-up. The longitudinal relationship throughout an illness trajectory becomes a cornerstone of pediatric palliative care. As more children with chronic illnesses survive into young adulthood, there is also an important role in transitioning to adult care teams. This can be challenging as many families have developed well-established relationships with pediatric providers.

1.6   Holistic Approach: Roles of Interdisciplinary Pediatric Palliative Care Team Members

Interdisciplinary pediatric palliative care teams are committed to complementarily addressing the physical, spiritual, and psychosocial needs of each child and family receiving care. Doing so requires ongoing clarification of skills, roles, resources, and team and individual priorities. More professional roles on a team increases the potential for creative problem-solving and holistic care, while also increasing the need for role clarity and time required for decision-making. A clear understanding of the roles of interdisciplinary pediatric palliative providers can help ensure effective use of these resources.

1.6.1   Pediatric Palliative Care Social Worker

Social work is defined as a helping profession by the National Association of Social Workers (NASW) with a commitment to advocacy, social justice, and supporting well-being and the needs of individuals, families, and communities. Social workers maintain diverse roles in a variety of settings or specialty areas, drawing upon practical experience and theoretical frameworks to perform within three interrelated levels of practice: micro (individual/family), mezzo (groups/organizations), and macro (large-scale systemic change).

The field of PPC social work continues to grow, and recently published definitions of core competencies (Jonas et al., 2022) delineate the specific skill base of PPC social workers in the following areas: specialized knowledge of palliative care in childhood, education, research, and quality improvement; advocacy; care planning and care delivery/clinical intervention; communication/information sharing; decision-making/advance care planning; family-centered care/family system; interprofessional team collaboration; evaluation/outcomes; program development; supervision and leadership; community capacity building; practical assistance (resource identification and referral); cultural responsiveness and antiracist action; self-care; well-being management; and reflective practice. Pediatric palliative care social workers have expertise in skilled psychosocial assessment; clinical consultation; brief therapeutic intervention; psychosocial and nonpharmacological approach to symptom management; concrete and practical resource assessment, referral, and advocacy; care coordination; anticipatory grief work; and bereavement care for a child with serious illness and their entire family. Alongside the interdisciplinary team, PPC social workers assist with complex medical decision-making. In addition, as defined by Jonas et al. (2022), they respond to and advocate for goals centered on personal and social roles and identities. Further, social workers assist a patient and their loved ones in adapting to and directly addressing disparities and challenges to their family, community, and cultural systems. PPC social workers also support clinicians and staff within their own health care institutions and PPC teams. The total number of PPC social workers nationally is not well documented, but in a survey of 162 PPC programs, 53.5% included a PPC social worker, typically in a position representing 0.5 of a full-time equivalent (Feudtner et al., 2013).

1.6.2   Pediatric Palliative Care Child Life Specialist

Certified child life specialists are health care professionals trained to provide psychosocial support to children and their families in various medical settings. While the specific support provided varies based on the unique patient and family needs, the overarching aim is to minimize the negative psychological effects that a hospitalization or difficult diagnosis can have on a child and their family. Examples of the types of assistance provided range from procedural support to help navigate the challenges that arise when a child is diagnosed with a chronic or life-limiting illness, including:

- Using developmentally appropriate language to prepare a child for a procedure or to explain a diagnosis
- Creating a coping plan to support a child through a procedure or treatment
- Using play to provide a child with a sense of control and normalcy
- Familiarizing a child with medical equipment through play
- Supporting the healthy development of coping skills and the expression of emotions through any combination of play, journaling, and other creative outlets
- Advocating for a child's right to have as much knowledge as they choose regarding their prognosis
- Assessing the needs of and providing support to siblings
- Guiding parents in discussing difficult news with their child(ren) in a developmentally appropriate way
- Providing opportunities for memory making and legacy building that include the creation of lasting mementos and memories
- Providing bereavement support at the end of a child's life

The integration of child life specialists into palliative care teams is relatively novel, with the first professional committee, Child Life Hospice and Palliative Care Network, being formed in 2022 (J. Mangers-Dean, personal communication, August 17, 2023). However, the American Academy of Pediatrics (2000) acknowledged the value of child life specialists in improving the quality of life of pediatric palliative care patients as early as 2000 and, more recently, recognized child life as an integral component of the palliative care team in providing end-of-life care (Linebarger et al., 2022).

1.6.3   Pediatric Palliative Care Chaplain

The palliative care chaplain is an integrated member of the palliative care team whose goal is to partner with team members to meet the spiritual and emotional needs of patients and families in both clinical and hospital settings. The chaplain uses different spiritual assessments depending on the spiritual, religious, cultural, or existential beliefs of a patient and family. Individuals can find themselves in spiritually or existentially challenging spaces within their own belief systems, based on what they are facing from a medical perspective. A chaplain will try to assess and address this existential crisis or advocate for a person's belief system by holding space and offering support. The ministry of presence is important in this space.

The palliative care chaplain is trained to offer spiritual and emotional support in clinical settings such as clinics, hospitals, and hospice facilities. Often a chaplain has completed Clinical Pastoral Education, is board certified, and has a master's or doctoral degree. This person is trained to offer unbiased support with cultural humility, grounded in a patient's spiritual understandings. In addition to patient support, the palliative care chaplain will also offer support for families, medical and non-medical staff, and caregivers based on needs assessed.

A palliative care chaplain offers compassionate listening, holding space for patients and families, asking open-ended questions, and advocating for the cultural, spiritual, and existential beliefs of patients and families. Palliative care chaplains can also administer spiritual rites or connect people with pastors/priests/ministers from the patient's belief systems in order to help with spiritual support. Palliative care chaplains are also often present near, or during, end of life to offer support for patients and families.

1.6.4   Pediatric Palliative Care Psychologist

Pediatric psychologists are doctoral-prepared providers with training in developmental psychology and psychopathology; social issues impacting youth and their families; evidence-based assessment, intervention strategies, and health promotion at the child, adolescent, and family levels; interdisciplinary team dynamics in care delivery; and research design, delivery, and evaluation (Palermo et al., 2014). These areas of competency highlight the unique skillsets that psychologists practicing in PPC contribute to the care of children and adolescents with serious illness and their families. For example, psychologists' expertise in psychosocial assessment assists the PPC team in determining whether a patient's or family member's state of mind and reactions during disease progression are normative, adaptive, or maladaptive, which then directly informs selection and implementation of empirically supported interventions—such as various breathing and relaxation techniques for symptom management and proven therapeutic approaches for alleviating emotional distress in both the patient and their family—aimed at reducing suffering, maintaining or improving quality of life, and supporting effective patient and family coping throughout the illness trajectory, including through end of life and into bereavement (Thompson et al., 2023).

A particularly valuable skillset possessed by well-trained psychologists is a comprehensive understanding of interdisciplinary psychosocial research methodology. In the PPC field, this entails the ability to navigate the challenges and ethical issues of research involving patients of diverse cognitive and physical abilities across various short- and long-term care settings (Thompson et al., 2023). Many psychologists are proficient in designing research protocols, adapting methodologies for implementation within specialty PPC services where necessary, and then analyzing and disseminating the results. A recent study showed that more than two-thirds of pediatric palliative care providers surveyed report a desire to have psychologists participate in their research because of their expertise in complex research design, advanced statistics, and scientific writing (Hildenbrand et al., 2021).

References

American Academy of Pediatrics (AAP). (2019). Clinical practice guidelines for quality palliative care. *Pediatrics, 143*(1), e20183310. https://doi.org/10.1542/peds.2018-3310

American Academy of Pediatrics, Committee on Bioethics and Committee on Hospital Care. (2000). Palliative care for children. *Pediatrics, 106*(2), 351–357. https://doi.org/10.1542/peds.106.2.351

Blume, E. D., Kirsch, R., Cousino, M. K., Walter, J. K., Steiner, J. M., Miller, T. A., Machado, D., Peyton, C., Bacha, E., Morell, E., & American Heart Association Pediatric Heart Failure and Transplantation Committee of the Council on Lifelong Congenital Heart Disease and Heart Health in the Young. (2023). Palliative care across the life span for children with heart disease: A scientific statement from the American Heart Association. *Circ: Cardiovascular Quality and Outcomes, 16*(2), e000114. https://doi.org/10.1161/HCQ.0000000000000114

Boland, L., Graham, I. D., Légaré, F., Lewis, K., Jull, J., Shephard, A., Lawson, M. L., Davis, A., Yameogo, A., & Stacey, D. (2019). Barriers and facilitators of pediatric shared decision-making: A systematic review. *Implementation Science, 14*(1), 7. https://doi.org/10.1186/s13012-018-0851-5

Clark, D. (2007). From margins to centre: A review of the history of palliative care in cancer. *The Lancet Oncology, 8*(5), 430–438. https://doi.org/10.1016/S1470-2045(07)70138-9

Delgado-Corcoran, C., Wawrzynski, S. E., Mansfield, K. J., Flaherty, B., DeCourcey, D. D., Moore, D., Cook, L. J., Ullrich, C. K., & Olson, L. M. (2022). An automatic pediatric palliative care consultation for children supported on extracorporeal membrane oxygenation: A survey of perceived benefits and barriers. *Journal of Palliative Medicine, 25*(6), 952–957. https://doi.org/10.1089/jpm.2021.0452

Feudtner, C., Womer, J., Augustin, R., Remke, S., Wolfe, J., Friebert, S., & Weissman, D. (2013). Pediatric palliative care programs in children's hospitals: A cross-sectional national survey. *Pediatrics, 132*(6), 1063–1070. https://doi.org/10.1542/peds.2013-1286

Harmoney, K., Mobley, E. M., Gilbertson-White, S., Brogden, N. K., & Benson, R. J. (2019). Differences in advance care planning and circumstances of death for pediatric patients who do and do not receive palliative care consults: A single-center retrospective review of all pediatric deaths from 2012 to 2016. *Journal of Palliative Medicine, 22*(12), 1506–1514. https://doi.org/10.1089/jpm.2019.0111

Harris, K. W., Ray, K. N., & Yu, J. (2023). Family caregivers of children with medical complexity: Changes in health-related quality of life and experiences of care coordination. *Academic Pediatrics, 1876–2859*(23), 00427–00428. Epub ahead of print. https://doi.org/10.1016/j.acap.2023.11.023.

Hildenbrand, A. K., Amaro, C. M., Gramszlo, C., Alderfer, M. A., Levy, C., Ragsdale, L., Wohlheiter, K., & Marsac, M. L. (2021). Psychologists in pediatric palliative care: Clinical care models within the United States. *Clinical Practice in Pediatric Psychology, 9*(3), 229–241. https://doi.org/10.1037/cpp0000402

Jonas, D., Patneaude, A., Purol, N., Scanlon, C., & Remke, S. (2022). Defining core competencies and a call to action: Dissecting and embracing the crucial and multifaceted social work role in pediatric palliative care. *Journal of Pain and Symptom Management, 63*(6), e739–e748. https://doi.org/10.1016/j.jpainsymman.2022.02.341

Katz, N. T., Hynson, J. L., & Gillam, L. (2021). Dissonance in views between parents and clinicians of children with serious illness: How can we bridge the gap? *Journal of Paediatrics and Child Health, 57*(9), 1370–1375. https://doi.org/10.1111/jpc.15612

Kaye, E. C., Smith, J., Zhou, Y., Bagatell, R., Baker, J. N., Cohn, S. L., Diller, L. R., Glade Bender, J. L., Granger, M. M., Marachelian, A., Park, J. R., Rosenberg, A. R., Shusterman, S., Twist, C. J., & Mack, J. W. (2023). Factors influencing parents' choice of palliative treatment goals for children with relapsed or refractory neuroblastoma: A multi-site longitudinal survey study. *Cancer*. Epub ahead of print. https://doi.org/10.1002/cncr.35149.

Kumar, A., & Allaudeen, N. (2016). To cure sometimes, to relieve often, to comfort always. *JAMA Internal Medicine, 176*(6), 731–732. https://doi.org/10.1001/jamainternmed.2016.1220

Lee, A., DeGroote, N. P., & Brock, K. E. (2023). Early versus late outpatient pediatric palliative care consultation and its association with end-of-life outcomes in children with cancer. *Journal of Palliative Medicine, 26*(11), 1466–1473. https://doi.org/10.1089/jpm.2023.0063

Linebarger, J. S., Johnson, V., Boss, R. D., & Section on Hospice and Palliative Medicine. (2022). Guidance for pediatric end-of-life care. *Pediatrics, 149*(5), e2022057011. https://doi.org/10.1542/peds.2022-057011

Moresco, B., & Moore, D. (2021). Pediatric palliative care. *Hospital Practice, 49*(Sup1), 422–430. https://doi.org/10.1080/21548331.2021.1964867

Palermo, T. M., Janicke, D. M., McQuaid, E. L., Mullins, L. L., Robins, P. M., & Wu, Y. P. (2014). Recommendations for training in pediatric psychology: Defining core competencies across training levels. *Journal of Pediatric Psychology, 39*(9), 965–984. https://doi.org/10.1093/jpepsy/jsu015

Rossfeld, Z. M., Miller, R., Fosselman, D. D., Ketner, A. R., Tumin, D., Tobias, J. D., & Humphrey, L. (2019). Timing of palliative consultation for children during a fatal illness. *Hospital Pediatrics, 9*(5), 373–378. https://doi.org/10.1542/hpeds.2018-0169

Rothschild, C. B., & Derrington, S. F. (2020). Palliative care for pediatric intensive care patients and families. *Current Opinion in Pediatrics, 32*(3), 428–435. https://doi.org/10.1097/MOP.0000000000000903

Schuetze, D., Ploeger, C., Hach, M., Seipp, H., Kuss, K., Bösner, S., Gerlach, F. M., van den Akker, M., Erler, A., & Engler, J. (2022). Care practices of specialized outpatient pediatric palliative care teams in collaboration with parents: Results of participatory observations. *Palliative Medicine, 36*(2), 386–394. https://doi.org/10.1177/02692163211065294

Sisk, B. A., Feudtner, C., Bluebond-Langner, M., Sourkes, B., Hinds, P. S., & Wolfe, J. (2020). Response to suffering of the seriously ill child: A history of palliative care for children. *Pediatrics, 145*(1), e20191741. https://doi.org/10.1542/peds.2019-1741

Thompson, A. L., Schaefer, M. R., McCarthy, S. R., Hildenbrand, A. K., Cousino, M. K., Marsac, M. L., Majeski, J., Wohlheiter, K., & Kentor, R. A. (2023). Competencies for psychology practice in pediatric palliative care. *Journal of Pediatric Psychology, 48*(7), 614–622. https://doi.org/10.1093/jpepsy/jsad007

Chapter 2
Pediatric Palliative Care Involvement in Specific Populations

2.1 Perinatal Palliative Care

With advances in the prenatal diagnosis of life-limiting fetal conditions through imaging technology and noninvasive testing, many families discover that their unborn child has major congenital anomalies with potentially serious and life-limiting sequelae before their child's delivery. They may face the decision to terminate the pregnancy (if services are legal and accessible) or to carry the pregnancy to term. When a pregnancy continues through delivery, parents may opt for aggressive medical management after birth, care focused solely on comfort, or initial resuscitation and deferred decision-making until more information is obtained postnatally. Perinatal palliative care is an emerging field that extends the principles of palliative medicine into the prenatal period to support families and fetuses/neonates from the time of suspected diagnosis through bereavement care.

Perinatal palliative care is the multicomponent provision of care for fetuses or neonates with a serious illness in the perinatal period (22 weeks gestation to 28 days after birth) and their parents, families, and involved health care providers, aimed to relieve pain and control symptoms and to improve the quality of care for and well-being of fetuses and infants and their families. It is holistic, family-centered, comprehensive, and multidimensional, so that it addresses not only the physical, but also psychological, social, and spiritual dimensions (Dombrecht et al., 2023). The 2019 statement from the American College of Obstetricians and Gynecologists (ACOG) underscores the importance of perinatal palliative care in providing compassionate support to families facing a life-limiting diagnosis for their unborn child or newborn. ACOG emphasizes the need for health care providers to offer comprehensive information about perinatal palliative care options, including pregnancy continuation, comfort care, and end-of-life support. The statement highlights the significance of patient-centered care, shared decision-making, and respect for families' values and preferences. ACOG also emphasizes interdisciplinary collaboration among health care professionals to ensure that families receive holistic care that addresses their physical, emotional, and spiritual needs throughout the perinatal period (ACOG, 2019).

Effective communication in perinatal palliative care involves clear and sensitive communication between health care providers and families, which is essential for establishing trust, addressing concerns, and facilitating shared decision-making. This underscores the importance of training health care professionals in communication skills and providing families with accurate and understandable information about their options.

2.1.1 Perinatal Palliative Care Teams

Central to the success of perinatal palliative care is the collaboration and expertise of a multidisciplinary team. The perinatologist or obstetrician plays a crucial role in the perinatal palliative care team. They are responsible for diagnosing fetal conditions, providing medical guidance, and facilitating discussions with the family regarding the prognosis and available options. The neonatologist is another essential member, particularly if the baby is born alive. They provide medical care to the newborn, manage symptoms, and coordinate care with other specialists as needed. Their expertise in neonatal medicine is invaluable in ensuring the comfort and well-being of the baby. A pediatric palliative care specialist brings expertise in symptom management, pain relief, and psychosocial support for both the baby and the family. They work closely with the neonatologist to develop a care plan that aligns with the family's goals and values, ensuring that every aspect of the baby's care is tailored to their individual needs. The role of the nurse is paramount in perinatal palliative care, providing hands-on care, education, and emotional support to the family throughout the pregnancy, birth, and beyond. A social worker addresses the emotional, financial, and logistical challenges that arise for families facing a life-limiting diagnosis. They provide counseling, connect families with community resources, and help facilitate difficult conversations about end-of-life care and bereavement support. Finally, spiritual care providers offer emotional and spiritual support, helping families navigate questions of faith, meaning, and purpose during this profoundly challenging time. They provide comfort and guidance, regardless of the family's religious beliefs or practices.

2.1.2 The Perinatal Palliative Care Consultation

In the prenatal period, the palliative care team collaborates with parents using shared decision-making to prepare a delivery plan addressing the goals of care for the neonate once he or she is born. This plan is an important way to communicate parents' values and the discussions that have occurred during pregnancy to the team of providers present during labor and delivery. Especially in cases of diagnostic uncertainty, it is important for parents to know that the plan can be altered based on their baby's status after birth; these contingencies can be addressed in the birth plan as well (English & Hessler, 2013). The process of delivery planning can be supportive and therapeutic as well as an important communication tool. It allows families to express their fears, values, hopes, and wishes. It also allows palliative care providers to communicate to medical teams these wishes for the rest of the pregnancy, the delivery, birth, and time after. This has been demonstrated to decrease maternal stress and promote family-centered care (Cortezzo et al., 2020).

A delivery plan should reflect the following key areas, though the format may vary:

- Identifying information (baby's name or the way in which he/she should be referred, parents' names, description of baby's medical condition)
- Anticipated labor/delivery process (support persons present, monitoring, mode of delivery, cord-cutting, lactation consultant)
- Desired interventions (extent of resuscitation, oxygen, suctioning, treatments for symptom management)
- Post-delivery care (feeding, bathing, spiritual requests, memory-making, location of care, autopsy, organ or tissue donation, mortuary)
- Subsequent care should the baby survive through hospital discharge (pediatrician, hospice referral, subspecialty care)
- Psychosocial support (sibling support, partner support, bereavement, religious or spiritual support)

In the neonatal period, perinatal palliative care teams can continue to support the parents/family with the shared decision-making process—information gathering; communication tailored to the parents' needs, values, and wishes; education about what different paths may look like; conflict resolution; and longitudinal support through the child's life.

Many teams also incorporate support for the health care providers—education about perinatal palliative care, formal and informal psychological support, and debriefings after death.

Perinatal palliative care programs can include a variety of components adapted to fit the specific needs of the setting where it is developed. Team structure may include any combination of medical and psychosocial support providers to meet the needs of the fetus/infant and their family as well as health care providers on both maternity and neonatal wards (Wool et al., 2016).

2.1.3 Potential Barriers to Providing Perinatal Palliative Care

Despite its importance, perinatal palliative care faces several barriers that may hinder its widespread provision. One significant challenge is the lack of awareness and understanding among health care providers and the public about perinatal palliative care options. This results in delayed or inadequate access to appropriate support for families facing a life-limiting diagnosis for their unborn child or newborn.

Furthermore, health care systems often lack standardized protocols and guidelines for perinatal palliative care, leading to variability in the quality and availability of services across different institutions and regions. Boan Pion et al. (2021) identified guideline awareness, additional training, and access to perinatal palliative care teams as satisfiers for health care professionals. A majority of health care providers expressed the need for perinatal palliative care guidelines (80%) and further palliative care training (94%) (Boan Pion et al., 2021). Inconsistency in guidelines and training can contribute to disparities in access to care based on factors such as geographic location, socioeconomic status, and cultural background.

Financial constraints also pose a barrier to providing perinatal palliative care as reimbursement policies may not adequately cover the comprehensive services required to support families throughout the perinatal period. This can limit the resources available for specialized medical interventions, psychosocial support, and bereavement services, further exacerbating the challenges faced by families during this difficult time.

Addressing these barriers requires concerted efforts to raise awareness, develop standardized guidelines, advocate for policy changes, and allocate sufficient resources to support the provision of perinatal palliative care. By overcoming these obstacles, health care providers can ensure that all families receive compassionate and comprehensive care when facing the diagnosis of a life-limiting condition in their unborn child or newborn.

2.2 Children with Heart Disease

The birth prevalence of congenital heart disease (CHD) has increased over time and presently affects ~8–10 per 1000 live births (van der Linde et al., 2011; Gilboa et al., 2016). Clinical advancements in the care of children with CHD have resulted in improved survival rates in this patient population, with >1 million children living with CHD in the United States (Gilboa et al., 2016; Blume et al., 2023; Bergsträsser et al., 2022). However, children living with CHD and advanced heart disease (AHD) are at risk of early mortality, disease trajectory uncertainty, and long-term comorbidities resulting in frequent hospitalizations with invasive interventions (Blume et al., 2023; Bergstrasser et al., 2022; Green et al., 2021). As such, this patient population needs the involvement of both primary palliative care and specialty palliative care (Blume et al., 2023; Bergstrasser et al., 2022). These services may be provided by the interdisciplinary cardiology team and complemented by the subspecialty-trained palliative care team on a consultative basis (Blume et al., 2023).

Studies have shown that pediatric palliative care (PPC) involvement in children with heart disease in a cardiac intensive care unit (CICU) occurs infrequently and late in the disease progression (Delgado-Corcoran et al., 2020; Green et al., 2021). The consultation usually occurs in the context of medical complexity and often close to the time of death rather than the time of diagnosis despite that a large proportion of children with congenital heart disease are diagnosed prenatally (Delgado-Corcoran et al., 2020; Green et al., 2021).

There is potential to increase palliative care consults in children in the CICU by standardizing the process of involving PPC, such as using screening criteria to identify patients who might benefit from a consultation. The Center to Advance Palliative Care (CAPC) has published criteria to identify children with heart disease who would be well served by a specialized palliative care consultation (Friebert & Osenga, 2022). These criteria may be used to prompt either a suggested or automatic consultation based on the complexity of heart disease, the presence of underlying neurologic or chromosomal diagnosis, frequency or duration of intensive care length of stay (>14 days), hospital length of stay (>3 weeks), and decision-making around the adoption of therapeutic technologies such as extracorporeal membrane oxygenation (ECMO), ventricular assist device, or organ transplantation (Friebert & Osenga, 2022).

Headrick et al. (2023) described the use of CICU length of stay of more than 14 days as screening criteria to identify patients eligible for a PPC consultation. The meeting of screening criteria was followed by a huddle between CICU staff members and PPC to determine the appropriateness of the consult. This quality improvement project resulted in a significant and clinically important increase in PPC consultation rates in a CICU where the rates of PPC consultation were traditionally low (Headrick et al., 2023). The use of screening criteria has the benefit of reducing the variability for who gets a PPC consultation and when. Pediatric CICUs would do well to emulate adult ICUs where the widespread use of screening criteria has led to increased palliative care consultation and decreased time to palliative care referral while reducing ICU resource utilization and improving the family and patient experience (Zalenski et al., 2017). Moynihan et al. (2019) described a champion-based model where designated CICU-based champions reinforce the PPC team through a variety of methods, including staff training, implementing quality improvement initiatives, and serving as a liaison between the PPC and CICU teams.

2.2.1 Benefits of Palliative Care Integration for Children with Heart Disease

The involvement of PPC consultation in children with heart disease is associated with improved quality of life, decreased hospital length of stay, and fewer invasive interventions at the end of life (Gilboa et al., 2016; Green et al., 2021; Delgado-Corcoran et al., 2020; Marcus et al., 2018). Among children with CHD and AHD, PPC consultation has been shown to support goal-concordant care that results in fewer deaths in the ICU during active resuscitation attempts, increased comfort care, and more deaths at home rather than in the hospital compared to children without PPC (Delgado-Corcoran et al., 2020; Marcus et al., 2018; Moynihan et al., 2021). As such, leading organizations, including the American Academy of Pediatrics (AAP) and the Improving Palliative Care in the Intensive Care Unit Advisory Board, recommend pediatric palliative care involvement at the time of diagnosis of a potentially life-limiting condition and continuing throughout disease trajectory, regardless of the outcome (Boss et al., 2014; AAP, 2014).

Referral at the time of diagnosis facilitates PPC involvement early in the disease trajectory, thus allowing the PPC team to build longitudinal relationships with patients and families throughout the duration of illness, facilitating early conversations about the goals of care and advance care planning (Moynihan et al., 2021). These relationships relieve patient and caregiver symptoms of pain, stress, anxiety, and depression while also providing end-of-life and bereavement support (Temel et al., 2017; El-Jawahri et al., 2017). A randomized trial in infants prenatally diagnosed with single-ventricle heart disease found that PPC referral prior to the first-stage palliative surgery was associated with decreased maternal anxiety and improved communication and family relationships (Hancock et al., 2018). Surveyed providers believe that prenatal PPC consults for patients with hypoplastic left heart syndrome provide a variety of benefits to families, including education, emotional support, and continuity of care (Lowenstein et al., 2020).

Overall, children with heart disease have highly intensive care at the end of life. However, involvement of PPC results in lower intensity of care and fewer interventions initiated in the last 14 days of life compared to those without PPC (Songer et al., 2023). The fact that children with heart disease have intense care at end of life regardless of PPC involvement suggests that goals of care of these families often align with pursuing life-prolonging treatment concurrently with the receipt of PPC (Marcus et al., 2018). This is in contrast to the perception that PPC consultation undermines parental hope or makes parents feel like the medical team is giving up, which is a barrier to PPC consultation elicited by cardiologists and pediatric cardiothoracic surgeons (Balkin et al., 2017).

2.2.2 Barriers and Facilitators to Palliative Care Integration for Children with Heart Disease

Despite the demonstrated benefits of palliative care in children with heart disease, there are barriers to its accessibility. Cardiologists worry about lack of benefit from PPC, involvement of new teams, fear of undermining parental hope, concerns that PPC will be poorly accepted by parents, and concerns that the philosophy of the palliative care team is inconsistent with provider therapeutic approach or that PPC only assists with end-of-life issues and is only appropriate for children who are dying or expected to die (Balkin et al., 2017). Pediatric congenital cardiothoracic surgeons also expressed concerns about the perceptions of "giving up" on the patient and of undermining parental hope (Morell et al., 2021). Unfortunately, there is a common misconception that PPC services are only useful for end-of-life care, or when all curative efforts have been exhausted, when, in fact, pediatric palliative care involvement works best when integrated with curative efforts early during the disease trajectory (Bogetz et al., 2014). Additionally, there is an unfamiliarity about the scope of practice of palliative care (Afonso et al., 2021). Barriers specific to the CICU include high prognostic uncertainty, availability of invasive technologies, and the focus on survival outcomes (Moynihan et al., 2021, 2019). Indeed, research indicates that, among children with CHD and AHD, PPC consultation often occurs later in the disease trajectory, suggesting that consultations do not occur until a time of crisis (Green et al., 2021; Marcus et al., 2018). While still beneficial, palliative care consultation in the context of crisis limits the ability of the PPC team to do what it does best—build a longitudinal relationship with families throughout the entire illness trajectory and ensure that the families' values, goals of care, and advance care planning are followed (Goloff & Joy, 2018).

Despite barriers to integrating PPC in children with heart disease, intensive care providers recognize that PPC helps facilitate multidisciplinary care conferences, assists with symptom management, and expertly navigates sensitive conversations, including end-of-life care discussions with families of critically ill children (Richards et al., 2018; Ciriello et al., 2018). Headrick et al. (2023) explored ICU providers' and families' perspectives toward PPC after the implementation of screening criteria to increase palliative care consultation in children with prolonged CICU stay. The project demonstrated that PPC is valued by CICU providers and families. CICU providers appreciate PPC involvement in supporting decision-making, identification of families' goals of care, decisions about end-of-life care, and psycho-spiritual support for families. Families stated that they value PPC in assisting with communication with the primary team, understanding their hopes and worries, and supporting their spiritual, psychological, and emotional needs (Headrick et al., 2023).

2.2.3   Conclusions

PPC consultation rates in children with heart disease are low and occur late in the disease trajectory. Consultation should be considered at the time of complex heart disease diagnosis either prenatally or postnatally in the presence of other comorbidities. Studies within the cardiac patient and provider populations have demonstrated that PPC is beneficial for the child, the family, and the care providers. More studies are warranted to evaluate how referral criteria can help connect families with PPC in a timely manner and measure the impact of PPC in the pediatric heart disease population.

2.3 Pediatric Oncology

2.3.1 Integration of Pediatric Palliative Care into Pediatric Hematology–Oncology Practice

Pediatric hematology–oncology (PHO) is a unique field that presents both opportunities and challenges for the pediatric palliative care provider. Cancer is both less commonly diagnosed and more likely to be successfully treated in children compared to adults (Siegel et al., 2023a). In the United States, approximately 15,190 children and adolescents from birth to 19 years were expected to be diagnosed with cancer in 2023, and 4.4% of all new cancers will be diagnosed in adolescents and young adults (15–39 years of age; Siegel et al., 2023b). Fortunately, most pediatric cancer patients are expected to become long-term survivors of their disease. Unfortunately, cancer remains the leading illness-based cause of death for children and adolescents, and multimodal cancer therapy often results in a host of acute and/ or chronic physical and psychological symptoms.

Pediatric palliative care aims to relieve suffering and improve the quality of life for children and their loved ones during disease-directed therapies and beyond, either into survivorship or to end-of-life care and parental bereavement (AAP, 2000). PHO is a field with clear palliative care overlap as patients are faced with serious life-threatening illnesses that may result in death, and they require sometimes painful, intensive, and high symptom-burden therapies for a chance at disease remission or cure. In fact, early integration of PPC principles and subspecialty palliative care services into the care of children with cancer is considered best clinical practice (Ferrell et al., 2018; Mack & Wolfe, 2006; Weaver et al., 2015; Kaye et al., 2016), yet implementation remains challenging due to provider beliefs (Hilden, 2016), concerns about parental hopes (Kaye et al., 2020; Levine et al., 2017), and limited availability of PPC practitioners/services.

Early integration of palliative care as a standard of care into oncology therapy allows for proactive identification of physical, social, spiritual, and psychological suffering within the patient and family context due to disease and its treatment (Ferrell et al., 2017, 2018; Weaver et al., 2015). PPC clinicians are experts in empathetic communication, and numerous studies have noted that parents of children with cancer perceive honest, clear communication as centrally important to their child's care (Contro et al., 2002; Kaye et al., 2021a, b). Palliative care has been shown to improve quality of life, decrease depressive symptoms, and improve patient outcomes for those with cancer (Temel et al., 2010). Palliative care can benefit pediatric cancer patients by decreasing physical symptoms and improving family preparedness for end of life (Wolfe et al., 2000b, 2008; Vern-Gross et al., 2015).

Pediatric palliative care providers need to understand several tenets within oncology practice to best synergize care with pediatric oncology providers. The National Hospice and Palliative Care Organization (NHPCO, 2022) identifies four diagnostic categories, based on disease characteristics, of the types of patients who should be afforded PPC services. Advanced or progressive cancer or cancer with a poor prognosis (along with severe congenital heart disease, trauma, sudden severe illness, or extreme prematurity) is designated as a Group 1 diagnostic category, which is defined as "life threatening conditions for which curative treatment may be feasible but can fail, where palliative care services may be beneficial alongside attempts at life-prolonging treatment and/or if treatment fails" (NHPCO, 2022). Cancer therapy can be difficult—symptoms from both the disease itself and from therapeutic modalities can negatively impact the quality of life, and many patients are willing to accept symptoms in pursuit of cure or even life prolongation. Oncology patients are typically cared for by a robust interdisciplinary team that provides wrap-around care for these patients and families. This team ideally begins to build relationships with a patient and family at diagnosis and follows closely throughout the disease trajectory, which can lead to friction at the introduction of a "new" supportive team if PPC is brought in later in the disease trajectory.

The oncology team must support the complex interplay between hope for cure and anticipation of potential mortality throughout the cancer trajectory (Wolfe et al., 2000a). Historically, PHO providers have worried that honest prognostic disclosure may lead to a decrease in parental hope, yet more recent work with cancer patients and their parents has shown this to be false (Kaye et al., 2020; Levine et al., 2017). In addition, some providers are at times hesitant to involve palliative care as they worry that patients/families "aren't ready yet." Provider concern regarding the timing of palliative care consultation has been disputed in surveys of patient/parent dyads whereby very few children (1.6%) or parents (6.2%) were opposed to the integration of a palliative care team at cancer diagnosis, and children with refractory symptoms were significantly more interested in palliative care involvement (Levine et al., 2017).

There are also times when a child has an incurable cancer but may not progress quickly to death. As the research and therapeutic options for high-risk cancers have evolved, there have been therapeutic developments that may allow more patients to live with cancer without the promise of permanent cure. These patients are a highly challenging area for palliative care as oncologists are often faced with delivering serious news regarding the incurability of a cancer and then immediately following this conversation with a discussion regarding further treatment options. This therapeutic uncertainty coupled with the toxic nature of many treatments requires providers to provide honest, empathetic communication with families to assure decision-making is family-centered and goal-directed. Research in this area shows that better prognostic understanding by the family and participation in advance care planning due to palliative care involvement lead to fewer reported symptoms, less suffering, and decreased parental regret after a child dies (Mack et al., 2015).

2.3.2 Benefits of Palliative Care Integration for Children with Cancer

Pediatric cancer patients who are involved with the pediatric palliative care team receive numerous benefits including improved symptom detection and management (Wolfe et al., 2008; Zhukovsky et al., 2009; Schmidt et al., 2013), improved coordination of care across settings (Zhukovsky et al., 2009), and more honest, timely communication (Kassam et al., 2015). Children and adolescents with cancer who have palliative care support are more likely to participate in advanced care planning to ensure that their care is goal directed (Weaver et al., 2015; Wolfe et al., 2008; Kassam et al., 2015). They also tend to have fewer hospital admissions and shorter lengths of stay (Fraser et al., 2013; Mitchell et al., 2017; Lo et al., 2022; Cheng & Wangmo, 2020). Cost savings for young people with cancer receiving palliative care were estimated to be $46,632 per hospitalization; mean daily savings were $1163 per day (Kaye et al., 2021c). Children with home-based palliative care services were found to have patient- and family-reported improvement in quality of life, and these children were more likely to die at home (Friedrichsdorf et al., 2015). Finally, children with cancer who are supported by PPC are more likely to enroll in hospice care and are less likely to die in the intensive care unit (Weaver et al., 2015; Wolfe et al., 2008; Snaman et al., 2017).

Symptom management expertise from PPC clinicians offers another unique and valuable benefit to PHO patients as the course of treatment may entail a significant symptom burden and contribute heavily to patient suffering (Levine et al., 2017). Additionally, there is a delicate interplay between a pediatric patient's well-being and the well-being of their parents/guardians. PPC involvement has been shown to improve the physical and mental health of pediatric patients' families due to more effective symptom management. Studies have shown a cause-and-effect cascade when delayed introduction of psychosocial support for patients and families leads to increased suffering and worsening symptoms, which correlate with impaired parental functioning (e.g., increased depressive symptoms and poorer coping in parents) (Olagunju et al., 2016; Ullrich et al., 2017).

In addition to a family's mental and physical well-being, communication is also improved with the addition of PPC services. Families who did not receive PPC services have been found to be at higher risk of not receiving critical end-of-life communication including anticipatory guidance about death and the dying process and preparation for the medical aspects surrounding their child's death (Kassam et al., 2015).

2.3.3 Potential Barriers to Palliative Care Integration for Children with Cancer

Despite the robust data proving substantial benefit, the early integration of palliative care services into pediatric cancer care remains challenging. Barriers may occur at multiple levels but have been categorized recently as (1) policy or payment barriers due to laws or insurer policies, (2) health system barriers such as workforce and access issues, (3) barriers due to organizational structure, culture, or policy, and (4) individual barriers due to beliefs, experiences, or resources of patients, families, and/or providers (Haines et al., 2018).

2.3.3.1 Policy and Payment Barriers

Many of the intensive psychosocial services required for these patients and families are historically under-reimbursed financially (Keim-Malpass et al., 2013). Unfortunately, coverage at times is dependent on local/regional policies, including state Medicaid, state waiver-based insurance plans, and/or access for those with private insurance plans, which can lead to inequities within or amongst regions (Haines et al., 2018). One way to address these barriers is to increase state funding and support/expansion of the Medicaid Concurrent Care for Children Requirement (Patient Protection and Affordable Care Act Section 2302), which would afford children the opportunity to be enrolled in concurrent hospice services without forgoing their current treatments within oncology. Concurrent hospice and therapeutic care supports families who often have blended goals of helping their child to live as long as possible (disease-directed or life-prolonging therapy) and to be as comfortable as possible (symptom- and comfort-focused care). In addition to expanding concurrent hospice services via state funding and support, the other option is to globally look at revising the hospice insurance benefit and removing the stipulation of "either-or" hospice or disease-directed therapy and instead offering the opportunity for patients, families, and children to gain hospice services without forgoing other treatments or relationships with their trusted care providers.

2.3.3.2 Workforce and Access Barriers

The availability of PPC teams has increased exponentially over the past several decades; however, most of the services rendered are in the inpatient or hospital setting, and some require philanthropic or grant-based funding to remain solvent (Haines et al., 2018). Staffing pediatric palliative teams, especially for 24/7 coverage, home-based support, and parental and sibling bereavement before and after the loss of a child can be challenging. Few pediatric-specific palliative care training programs exist, and special expertise is required to care for pediatric cancer patients nearing the end of life. Pediatric oncology providers are increasingly likely to pursue primary palliative care education, yet palliative education is not a requirement for pediatric oncology fellowship graduation or practice (Baker et al., 2007). In response, the field of pediatric palliative oncology has been developed to meet the specific needs of children with cancer (Snaman et al., 2020; Kaye et al., 2016). Unique dual programs have been created to train subspecialty providers with expert-level skills in both disciplines; however, dual-trained clinicians remain sparse, which emphasizes the importance of pediatric palliative care provider willingness and knowledge to care for these complex patients with oncologic diagnoses (Snaman et al., 2020).

In the ideal balance between primary and subspecialty pediatric palliative care, most primary palliative care is provided by pediatric oncology clinicians, while subspecialty palliative care is reserved for refractory symptom management and family-centered communication surrounding grief, anticipatory guidance at end of life, and advanced care planning. Targeted engagement with the limited resource of subspecialty palliative care is an important consideration and allows for a focus on specific areas where there is a high need such as those recommended by CAPC (2022), including diffuse intrinsic pontine glioma, stage IV neuroblastoma, metastatic solid tumors, any other cancer with projected 5-year event-free survival <40% with currently available therapies, new diagnosis with complex pain or other symptom management issues, and any disease in which hematopoietic stem cell transplantation is part of the upfront treatment plan.

2.3.3.3 Organizational Structure, Culture, and Policy Barriers

Barriers also stem from complex care management across multiple settings and provider groups. In fact, the palliative care consultative model requires that an oncology provider must be aware of the PPC team and understand the palliative care benefits for their patient before a consultation can even be placed. Adding a PPC team to an already complex management situation can be beneficial to the patient and family while also complicating the care received by the patient. In addition, due to workforce and reimbursement issues described above, the PPC team is involved with only a fraction of the oncology patients at an institution.

2.3.3.4 Individual Patient/Provider Barriers

Barriers reported in the literature (pertaining primarily to clinical practice in the United States) include PHO clinician perceptions that families "aren't ready" for specific prognostic or goal-directed conversations (Hilden, 2016). A growing body of literature, however, details parent and patient acceptance of early integration of PPC into the care plan.

Oncologists and the interdisciplinary oncology teams often believe they are providing a high degree of support and care for children with serious illness and may resist engagement with another interdisciplinary team (Humphrey & Kang, 2015). Oncologists may also lack knowledge or have underlying beliefs about the utility of pediatric palliative care for their patients, and they may believe that concurrent goals of cure and comfort are at odds (Dalberg et al., 2013). As palliative care has become an increasingly broad discipline serving to improve quality of life regardless of the trajectory of a disease, the myths equating palliation to hospice or comfort support are dissipating, yet this belief may still dictate practice for some providers (Haines et al., 2018). Barriers may stem not only from medical providers, but also from providers of psychosocial supportive services on the primary oncologic care team who may have concerns surrounding therapeutic relationships and/or duplicative services when additional supportive teams are consulted (Dalberg et al., 2013). Finally, as the supportive services of a palliative care team are often stretched across the hospital system, it is difficult to meet the acute and immediate needs of all potential patients in oncology; thus, equitable early engagement often is not possible for all patients with the same diagnosis.

Patients and families may have similar misgivings or misconceptions about palliative care equating to end-of-life care. This is especially true when the patient is referred late in their illness (Haines et al., 2018). When patients have few options for cancer-directed therapy and are unlikely to be cured, some families have difficulty both pursuing additional chemotherapy while engaging with the palliative care team, though evidence shows that PPC can foster hope rather than take it away (Kaye et al., 2020; Baker et al., 2008). Despite these anecdotal parent concerns, most parents are incredibly open to early integration of PPC into cancer care when it is defined as holistic support for the patient and family (Levine et al., 2017).

Cultural barriers can also pose challenges to the integration of the PPC team, including beliefs about how to involve children in diagnosis and treatment, who should be the primary decision-makers for a child with cancer, and how and when to talk to children about their imminent death. Through shared decision-making, both the oncologist and palliative care clinicians can work to de-stigmatize PPC and operate from patient- and family-identified goals of care and definition of quality of life.

2.3.4   Palliative Care Integration Opportunities for Stem Cell Transplantation

Hematopoietic stem cell transplant (HSCT) is an intensive, primarily inpatient therapy that seeks to provide curative options for children with certain cancers and other diagnoses. With HSCT, the symptom burden can be quite high, with a substantial risk of both acute and long-term problems and/or death. Data for adolescent and young adult patients post HSCT who subsequently died compared with non-HSCT oncology patients showed that the HSCT group was more likely to die in the ICU, receive mechanical ventilation, and undergo hemodialysis in the last 30 days of life (Snaman et al., 2018). The barriers to PPC engagement in HSCT are similar to those in PHO in general, while this patient population in particular may elicit significant benefits with collaborative engagement. With the high potential benefit of having a PPC consultation, it is also an area worth investigating as a trigger criterion.

2.3.5   The Future of Pediatric Oncology and Palliative Care

As training opportunities expand and oncologists seek additional education in palliative care, there are opportunities for embedding palliative care physicians in oncology teams across the country.

New symptom measurements are validated in pediatric oncology practice to include the Patient Reported Outcomes for Common Terminology for Cancer Toxicity Events (PRO-CTCAE; National Cancer Institute, 2023). The CTCAE scoring rubric is used in most oncology trials to denote grading of side effects from a provider perspective; however, the PRO-CTCAE is a patient report of symptom outcomes, and the pediatric version is now available free of charge through the National Cancer Institute for use in pediatric trials. Incorporation of these symptom scores into the clinical care of PHO patients and as trial metrics will provide the most reliable information about symptom prevalence, severity, and duration, as well as feedback on the management of symptoms, offering oncologists new opportunities to engage with PPC teams and evaluate the effectiveness of symptom management.

Expansion of concurrent hospice and therapeutic care services may also broaden the reach of palliative care teams to patients with oncologic diagnoses, which could impact the potential for added symptom management opportunities in the home setting, decreased emergency room visits and hospitalizations, and perhaps a higher percentage of patients with end-stage cancer who have the opportunity to die at home instead of in the hospital.

Close partnerships between oncology teams and palliative care teams also offer earlier engagement, bilateral team growth to meet the expanding needs of patients, and opportunities for added engagement in the setting of chronic cancer syndromes (e.g., patients living with cancer for years without remission or progression).

2.3.6   Conclusions

Pediatric palliative care and pediatric oncology teams have promising opportunities to collaborate in the holistic care of children with oncologic diagnoses. Pediatric cancer patients and families involved with PPC experience measurable benefits in symptom management, anticipatory guidance/advance care planning, coping, mental/physical health, and communication. There are still barriers to engaging PPC teams even as the workforce develops and as stigmatization of PPC as relevant only to hospice and end-of- life care declines. With new and evolving treatments, technologies, and modalities, more children are living with chronic cancer diagnoses and undergoing treatments with higher potential complications and symptom burden, as in bone marrow transplantation, which offer new opportunities to partner with PPC. The hope of many patients, families, and providers is that as PPC evolves as a field, access and equity will improve and there will be more opportunities to engage earlier during the diagnosis and treatment of pediatric oncologic diseases.

2.4 Pediatric Neurology

Many patients with neurological conditions face chronic symptom burdens, limited treatment options, and unpredictable trajectories, making them good candidates for palliative care support. Benefits of PPC involvement for patients with neurological diagnoses include (1) support with symptom management, (2) psychosocial and spiritual support for families facing long-term and variable prognoses, (3) longitudinal goals of care and advance care planning discussions, and (4) end-of-life support, including hospice and bereavement services for parents and siblings. However, barriers to effective PPC integration with neurology exist, including (1) how to determine when specialty palliative care offers value in addition to the primary palliative care provided by neurologists, (2) when to refer patients with variable disease courses, and (3) the absence of disease-specific palliative guidelines for pediatric neurological disorders (Lyons-Warren et al., 2019).

2.4.1 Palliative Care Involvement in Children with Primary Neurological Diagnoses

The American Academy of Neurology formally recognized the need for neurologists to use the principles of palliative medicine in 1996, and since then, the adult and pediatric neurology communities have consistently validated the importance of palliative care involvement for patients with neurological diagnoses (Borasio, 2013; Provinciali et al., 2016). Estimates of the percentage of children with primary neurological diagnoses receiving palliative care are limited in the literature. However, existing data suggests that referrals for primary neurological disorders are common in PPC. At our institution, a tertiary care children's hospital in the Intermountain West, from January 2007 to October 2021, 452 patients with a primary neuromuscular diagnosis were referred to PPC (16% of total referrals), and 1157 patients with a genetic or congenital syndrome were referred (42% of total referrals), many of which have a primary neurological problem. In a pediatric multicenter study of 515 palliative care patients, genetic (40.8%) and neuromuscular (39.2%) diagnoses were common, suggesting significant use of palliative services by patients with neurological conditions (Feudtner et al., 2011).

2.4.2 Palliative Care for Infants with Neurological Diagnoses

Infants with neurological disorders present unique challenges for the PPC and neurology teams as new diagnoses, unexpected clinical courses, and the need for discussions about prognosis are particularly stressful for families of newborns. Each diagnosis has its own considerations, including infants with neuromuscular disorders that may require long-term feeding or respiratory support, hypoxic encephalopathy with profound brain injury, severe structural brain abnormalities such as lissencephaly and genetic epilepsies to name a few. These families may benefit from meeting with PPC early to start to consider prognosis and treatment options and to delineate goals that impact the patient and family.

2.4.3 Benefits of Palliative Care for Children with Neurological Diagnoses

Addressing issues related to quality of life for patients with lifelong neurological conditions is a fundamental part of high-quality care (Defanti & Ad Hoc Working Group of the Italian Neurological Society, 2000). For neurology patients with chronic illness, palliative care involvement has been associated with improved symptom management. Failure to utilize a palliative care specialist contributes to worse control for both physical and cognitive symptoms, along with an increase in physical and emotional distress for the patient and the family (Dallara et al., 2014). While no prospective or randomized controlled studies have evaluated the impact of palliative care involvement specifically in pediatric neurology patients in the intensive care setting, one study based in a neonatal intensive care unit, including patients hospitalized for primary neurological issues, found that palliative care involvement increased the frequency of redirection of care when this aligned with parent goals, as well as increased do-not-resuscitate orders (Younge et al., 2015). Examples of effective integration of palliative care in neurology can be seen in neuromuscular clinics, which also tend to be interdisciplinary (Ho & Straatman, 2013). Finally, parents of children with neurological diagnoses, especially severe neurological impairment, have often reported feeling isolated as they face significant caregiving burdens, even when their child's disease process is relatively stable (Steele, 2000; Bogetz et al., 2021). Parents have expressed the feeling that they are the only ones who understand their child's holistic picture and that it can be burdensome to frequently repeat information and coordinate with other subspecialists (Bogetz et al., 2021). Palliative care providers are well suited to support these communication and psychosocial needs (Hauer & Wolfe, 2014).

2.4.4 Barriers to Palliative Care Involvement for Children with Neurological Diagnoses

While there is significant support for early integration of PPC in patients with primary neurological diagnoses (Oliver et al., 2016), several barriers still exist. First, many neurologists may feel comfortable providing some primary palliative care and feel unclear about when to refer for specialist support. Second, for patients with unpredictable trajectories or extended periods of stability, it can be difficult to determine the optimal time for PPC involvement. There may also be institutional barriers to collaboration. A survey of neurology and palliative care teams from six sites in the United Kingdom showed that a minority (36%) of neurologists reported "good or excellent" collaboration with palliative care services (Hepgul et al., 2018), and another study found that some neurologists expressed confusion about how to effectively integrate the interdisciplinary palliative team with the neurology service (Vanopdenbosch et al., 2017). Additionally, while disease-specific guidelines for palliative care involvement exist for some adult neurological disorders, these do not exist in pediatrics. Research to help define PPC referral metrics for pediatric neurology patients is needed. Finally, misconceptions about palliative care, such as equating it with giving up or exclusively applying to end-of-life scenarios, create barriers to palliative involvement in many specialties, including neurology.

2.4.5   Conclusion

Pediatric patients with primary neurological diagnoses face uncertain prognosis, limited life expectancy, high symptom burden, and demanding roles for caregivers. They benefit from frequent and evolving conversations around goals of care and may benefit from hospice involvement at the end of life. The literature demonstrates the benefit of PPC in settings such as the ICU and neuromuscular clinics, but gaps exist in terms of better integrating PPC more broadly. Understanding the benefits and roles of interdisciplinary PPC providers can support the appropriate use of palliative services for patients with primary neurological diagnoses.

2.5   Children and Youth with Special Health Care Needs

Children and youth with special health care needs (CYSHCN) are described by the Health Resources and Services Administration's Maternal and Child Health Bureau (MCHB, 2022) as "those who have or are at increased risk for a chronic physical, developmental, behavioral, or emotional condition and who also require health and related services of a type or amount beyond that required by children generally." Much has been learned about this population through the annual National Survey of Children's Health (NSCH) conducted by the United States Census Bureau (Ghandour et al., 2022). The survey is sent to US households and is completed by parents or guardians regarding young people living in the home. Data from the 2019 to 2020 survey period indicate that 14.1 million children (or 19.4% of young people) in the United States were designated as CYSHCN (Health Resources and Services Administration MCHB, 2022). Use of the screening tool with families in Europe yielded similar rates of prevalence (Davis et al., 2015). The designation of CYSHCN is broad and includes young people diagnosed with asthma, autism spectrum disorder, ADD/ADHD, Tourette syndrome, brain injury, epilepsy, genetic conditions, and cystic fibrosis, among others (Davis et al., 2015). Factors considered in designation as CYSHCN include use of prescription medications, functional limitations, and service utilization (medical, education, behavioral health) (Ghandour et al., 2022). The community of CYSHCN includes young people with a wide variety of diagnoses, prognoses, life expectancies, and illness effects, not all of whom have need for PPC. Those with significant service utilization and/or functional limitations often benefit from PPC involvement.

2.5.1 Children with Medical Complexity

Children with medical complexity, a subgroup of CYSHCN, are identified by prolonged and/or frequent hospitalizations, intensive service needs, technology/medical support dependence (e.g., ventilator use, gastrostomy feeding, dialysis), and increased care coordination needs (Cohen et al., 2011; Kuo et al., 2016). An estimated 320,000–1,200,200 children meet this description, representing 0.4–1.6% of the total population of children in the United States (Warren et al., 2022). It has been noted that this population has increased over the last 20 years, attributable to improved treatments and survival for conditions such as prematurity and congenital diseases, as well as improvements in acute care delivery (Cohen et al., 2011; Zorko et al., 2023). Children with medical complexity are estimated to utilize one-third of health care spending for all children in the United States (Kuo et al., 2016).

The 2022 MCHB Guiding Principles for services to CYSHCN include four areas of priority: "health equity, family and child well-being and quality of life, access to services and supports, and financing of services" (Warren et al., 2022). Families of children with medical complexity often navigate multiple subspecialist appointments and recommendations, medications, supplies, and education advocacy in addition to direct care needs. Unexpected events such as hospitalizations, changes in home nursing or school staffing, or acute illness can tax already limited resources. The segment of the CYSHCN population that is most often referred to pediatric palliative care includes those facing such obstacles given the field's emphases on family support and education, care coordination, supported decision-making, and symptom management.

2.5.2 Disparities Affecting Children and Youth with Special Health Care Needs

Given that quality of life and family support are essential considerations in palliative care, providers must practice with knowledge of social circumstances' effects upon the course of illness. Further, providers need to understand that disparities can increase disease burden by creating barriers to helpful treatments or supports. Important disparities affect the CYSHCN community (Ghandour et al., 2022; Warren et al., 2022). Families of CYSHCN have higher rates of poverty and receipt of public assistance (Warren et al., 2022; Schiff et al., 2022). CYSHCN living in poverty have higher rates of disability, and those with disability have increased unmet needs, decreased access to services, and lower likelihood of receiving care in well-run systems (Houtrow et al., 2022). Families in disadvantaged circumstances will benefit from PPC's targeted advocacy for high-quality care, early identification of unmet needs, and care coordination to avoid or delay disability. In terms of race and ethnicity, children and youth identified as having special health care needs are less likely to be Hispanic or non-Hispanic Asian, and fewer families with both parents born outside of the United States, or for whom English is not the primary language, report having children with special health care needs. These findings raise concern that Hispanic and Asian children may be under-identified (Ghandour et al., 2022). Providers should be vigilant for these patients who may not self-identify as having special needs but who would be best served by PPC involvement. In order to promote equitable patterns of referral to palliative care services, providers can utilize supports such as consult triggers.

2.5.3   Specialized Support for Children and Youth with Special Health Care Needs and Their Families

Types of need among CYSHCN vary widely by medical condition, with families requiring varying degrees of legal, educational, medical/dental, social, basic need, or advocacy support (Roman et al., 2020; Graaf & Gigli, 2022). Available PPC services for families dealing with serious illness may address care coordination, financial impact, or social needs associated with care. The benefits of informed, efficient care coordination have been illustrated, including decreasing rates of disparity and unmet needs (Roman et al., 2020). Unmet needs noted in literature include specialized care such as speech, occupational, and physical therapies, durable medical equipment, home health care, and mobility aids (Graaf & Gigli, 2022). Home health is particularly important as an estimated 1.5 billion hours of care for CYSHCN are attributed to family caregivers each year (Warren et al., 2022). For many families of CYSHCN, the cost of care and insurance coverage is also a major concern. As medical costs are often sizeable and unpredictable, appropriate payment systems are critical (Schiff et al., 2022). NSCH data from 2016 to 2019 show that a significant portion of surveyed families considered their insurance coverage inadequate or were entirely without coverage (Schiff et al., 2022).

Many programs and policies exist to help address the varied and unique needs of CYSHCN and their families. These range from the Katie Beckett provision of the Tax Equity and Fiscal Responsibility Act of 1982, which can be used by families to fund home care (Warren et al., 2022; Graaf & Gigli, 2022), and the Patient Protection and Affordable Care Act, which offers various coverage protections and benefits such as expansion of Medicaid and the elimination of lifetime benefit maximums and preexisting condition exclusions (Warren et al., 2022), to countless local, national, and international organizations that serve to connect families for shared wisdom, emotional and social support, and additional resources. Pediatric palliative care social workers can educate families on applicable programs and offer essential support as they navigate eligibility, application, usage, and renewal processes.

2.5.4   Conclusion

Millions of children and young adults in the United States have special health care needs. Disparities exist in the identification of, and thereby service to, children in some groups. Approximately one million CYSHCN have complex medical needs that require resource-intensive and specialized medical attention, coordination, and family support. Given the longitudinal, multisetting, and multidisciplinary nature of pediatric palliative care, it is well suited to support families of young people in these circumstances.

2.6   Adolescent and Young Adult Patients

The term adolescent and young adult (AYA) refers to patients making the transition from childhood to adulthood. The parameters for this group vary among organizations. AYA is defined by the National Cancer Institute (2024) as patients ages 15–39 years. The movement to transition patients from pediatric to adult models of care often uses the term AYA to refer to patients ages 11–25. Given the focus on the shift from one care setting to another, it is also useful to refer to this population as "transitional" patients. In this section, we will review PPC capabilities that are particularly relevant to this general population.

Distinction of the AYA and transitional population is important. A common principle is the recognition that the transition from pediatric to adult care is filled with tasks, challenges, and opportunities unlike any others. Outcomes are often poorer, with a relative lack of clinical trials to promote best evidence-based medical practice (Ferrari et al., 2021). For patients with chronic conditions, this period is often associated with difficulty adhering to treatment plans, leading to exacerbation of chronic illnesses. Higher acute care utilization rates, health costs, and morbidity are all seen to varying degrees during this transitional period (Jarvis et al., 2021; Parsons et al., 2023; Wurm et al., 2022).

2.6.1   Adolescent Brain Development

Adolescence is a developmental phase—a time of change and challenge. Physical changes (growth spurts), hormonal changes (puberty), and behavioral changes combined can make this especially challenging. For PPC teams, knowing the biological and developmental underpinnings of adolescence can assist them in helping seriously ill adolescents understand and cope with their illness. It is also very helpful for PPC providers to understand this developmental phase so that they, in turn, can help other providers better care for their adolescent patients.

Greater amygdala activation in adolescents than in adults (the degree of which varies across socioeconomic situations) suggests that adolescents can be hyperreactive in their responses to emotional stimuli; they tend to be less capable of regulating their own emotions and responding maturely to difficult situations (Jetha & Segalowitz, 2012). The adolescent brain (age 14–16 years) responds similarly to both pain and social exclusion, more so than child or adult brains. Physical changes related both to puberty and to illness and/or treatment can alter how adolescents see themselves and their perception of how others see them, and this sensitivity to social interactions can cause these changes to lead to concerns around body image and self-worth, exacerbating the adolescent's experience of total pain.

Self-regulating and executive functions are still developing in the prefrontal cortex. Add in the stressors of illness (uncomfortable symptoms, psychosocial factors, family dynamics, etc.), and the adolescent may be prone to impaired choices and behaviors. In the setting of immature self-regulation, there is an increase in dopamine reward pathways in the brain, thereby heightening responsiveness to reward stimuli, especially food, social stimuli, and novelty. This can lead to increased risk-taking and stimuli-seeking behaviors, including alcohol and drug use. Adolescents with chronic health care conditions are also more likely to suffer from disordered eating, and practitioners should be especially vigilant in screening for it in this population (Kumar, 2023). Adolescents also have more emphasis on short-term rewards rather than long-term goals or consequences (Jetha & Segalowitz, 2012), which may further result in immature decision-making and can affect treatment adherence.

These are just a few of the behaviors or changes that are seen in adolescents that may affect the way they cope with their illness and treatment efforts. All this biological change is laid on top of a foundation of personality, early childhood experiences, environment, and genetics. In light of this, it is important not to generalize, to approach each adolescent or young adult as an individual, and to not make assumptions (Straehla et al., 2017; Jetha & Segalowitz, 2012). After all, the human brain is complex, and many adolescents respond to stress and emotion as well as or better than adults.

2.6.2 Adolescent and Young Adult Needs

To provide the best care to patients, especially where psychosocial support services may be limited, PPC providers have to understand the needs of their patients. Several studies have sought to understand AYA and transitional needs. AYA patients report growth and sources of strength in existing relationships, future plans/goals, health competence, and spirituality/religious beliefs as most important for their sense of well-being (Bellizzi et al., 2012; Straehla et al., 2017). Connection to other adolescents and young adults with chronic illnesses, as in AYA patients with cancer, is also reported to foster well-being (Pulewka et al., 2021; Allen et al., 2022). AYA patients with cancer have expressed that the following domains were negatively impacted by their illness: finances, body image, control over life, work plans, fertility/family planning, and dating. Health care providers can underestimate the importance of these issues. In some studies, oncology providers significantly underestimated the need for sexual, fertility, mental health, employment/education, and body image counseling/support in AYA patients. Physical therapy, complementary and alternative medicine, and access to social work are other areas where the AYA population has been historically underserved (Kirchhoff et al., 2017). Studies assessing needs are ongoing as health care providers work on better understanding how to best treat these patients and improve current outcomes (Smith et al., 2018; Kirchhoff et al., 2017). PPC providers can help bridge this gap between what adolescents really want and what their health care providers think is most important.

2.6.3 Sexuality and Reproduction

The World Health Organization (WHO, n.d.) states that sexual health encompasses wide-ranging issues, including sexual orientation and gender identity, sexual expression, relationships, and pleasure. This definition also includes negative consequences or conditions such as sexually transmitted infections, sexual dysfunction, and sexual violence, among others (Reinman et al., 2021; WHO, n.d.). Establishing a sexual identity and positive body image are often milestones achieved during adolescence and young adulthood and can be disrupted by serious illness. It is important for providers to screen for these issues as adolescents report they are more likely to discuss their concerns if the provider brings it up first (Albers et al., 2022).

Body image issues, especially at a time when others' perceptions change and become more important to the adolescent, can be difficult. Disfigurement, nutritional problems, and other concerns all contribute to 60% of AYA and transitional patients having body image issues, potentially affecting relationships and sexuality (Kirchhoff et al., 2017; Allen et al., 2022; Wurm et al., 2022).

Many AYA patients report not fully understanding fertility issues until they pursue parenthood, when fear of not being able to conceive can cause psychological distress (Bellizzi et al., 2012; WHO, n.d.; Greenzang et al., 2020). Most patients benefit from discussing the goals for family and future relationships early; unfortunately, those goals are not always addressed. One study showed that only 34% of female AYA patients said they discussed their fertility preservation with a health care provider before their cancer treatment compared with 70% of male AYA patients (Shnorhavorian et al., 2015). Lately, awareness of this population and fertility concerns has improved, but data regarding patients' perceptions and outcomes is lacking (Klijn et al., 2023; Perez et al., 2020; Kirchhoff et al., 2017). PPC providers often have longitudinal relationships with their patients and can address fertility issues at the beginning of treatment, as well as throughout care (Greenzang et al., 2020).

In exploring these themes, it is important to note that AYA and transitional patients have their own individual experience, and many may not worry about any of this. Approaching these issues requires communication skills that focus on eliciting patient preference, responding to emotion, and coming to a shared decision. The PPC interdisciplinary team is often best positioned to address these concerns. The most important thing that providers can do is to approach sexual health issues in a normalizing, nonjudgmental way and treat adolescents and young adults with chronic health conditions with the same sexual health screening and anticipatory guidance that all adolescents should receive (Albers et al., 2022; WHO, n.d.).

2.6.4 Psychological Support

Up to 20% of children with chronic health conditions are reported to have significant psychological distress (Kirchhoff et al., 2017). The incidence of psychological disorders naturally increases in the AYA age group and, as with sexual health, clinicians should screen for these disorders (Jetha & Segalowitz, 2012; WHO, 2021).

Anxiety is prevalent among AYA and transitional patients with various dissimilar chronic conditions (Kirchhoff et al., 2017; Wurm et al., 2022; AAP, 1993). Youth with sickle cell disease report worsened anxiety and depression compared to peers; those with systemic lupus erythematosis have increased feelings of self-consciousness. Individuals with neurofibromatosis type 1 reported decreased quality of life with more emotional and behavioral problems (Allen et al., 2022). And patients tend to report guilt for family distress during and due to their illness (Perez & Greenzang, 2019).

Limited or nonexistent access to psychological support is one barrier to optimal care for these patients. The varied developmental stages, psychosocial concerns, and transitional age of care (whether seeking care in the adult or pediatric world) may all lead to decreased access to the highest quality care in part due to providers and health care systems not recognizing the diverse needs of this population (Hoegy et al., 2022; McGrady & Pai, 2019). PPC teams can supplement this psychological and social support for patients and families.

2.6.5 Palliative Care for AYA and Transitional Patients: Where Palliative Care Adds Value

Much has been said and valuable information exists regarding the transition from the pediatric world to the adult world. Fewer resources are available for adults (>21 years) in the pediatric arena, where their developmental stage has significantly surpassed the traditional demographic. Many pediatric centers have minimal experience in treating patients with a history of substance use disorder or patients with autonomy and complex social issues, actively pursuing advance care planning, or treating total body pain versus physical-only pain (Humphrey & Dell, 2015). PPC can be a bridge between the pediatric and adult world, with providers trained in both populations and having experience in many of these potentially challenging situations (Humphrey & Dell, 2015; Sansom-Daly, 2023). Pediatric palliative care is particularly well poised to assist in three main areas of difficulty for the AYA population, discussed below: treatment adherence, multiple and potentially confusing transition situations, and goal establishment and concordance.

2.6.5.1 Treatment Adherence

The reasons for AYA and transitional nonadherence to treatment are as varied and diverse as the population, with reported rates of nonadherence as high as 30–50% (higher than child and older adult nonadherence rates) (McGrady & Pai, 2019). In cancer, nonadherence rates of even 5% can lead to an increased risk of relapse (Newman & Hunger, 2023). In sickle cell disease, transitional patients have decreased adherence to treatments and appointments, leading to increased utilization of acute care and worse pain control (Hoegy et al., 2022). Nonadherence rates have no concordance with disease type, demographic variables (age, gender, race, socioeconomic status, religion, educational or occupational status, parental education status, family composition), or cognitive abilities, making it hard for providers to develop prediction models (Carr & Rosengarten, 2021; McGrady & Pai, 2019). There is limited data on this topic, but the research that does exist shows these factors all contribute to adherence rates: self-efficacy, ability to think about long-term consequences, environment, resources (family, access to psychological support, etc.), physical function, and symptoms (McGrady & Pai, 2019).

Providers, especially adult providers, can become frustrated with AYA and transitional patients' apparent lack of self-efficacy. However, that apparent lack of autonomy in adolescents and young adults can be developmentally appropriate when dealing with the stress of a serious illness. Members of a PPC interdisciplinary team are well suited to assist with this aspect of AYA and transitional patient care by educating primary care providers and parents on AYA developmental stages and needs. Providing this insight can help bridge therapeutic divides (Carr & Rosengarten, 2021; Jetha & Segalowitz, 2012) and encourage greater parental involvement, which leads to some of the highest levels of adherence in the younger members of this cohort (Carr & Rosengarten, 2021; Sonneveld et al., 2013). Additionally, continued check-ins, approached with a curious and nonjudgmental mindset, can build rapport and trust (McGrady & Pai, 2019). When clinicians do not regularly check in with open discussions, trust does not build, and opportunities are missed to improve health and treatment adherence. The PPC team provides those important longitudinal check-in opportunities with clinicians skilled in communication.

One specific area of nonadherence is difficulty in understanding the role of maintenance therapy: adolescents think, "If I feel good why take the medication?" (Carr & Rosengarten, 2021). Asymptomatic individuals who miss medication may doubt what professionals tell them; they are not always able to process the long-term risks since short-term outcomes can be more influential on the adolescent brain. PPC providers can provide increased psychological support and the positive reinforcement adolescents need to achieve better behavioral learning and reach treatment goals (Carr & Rosengarten, 2021; Jetha & Segalowitz, 2012). For patients whose diseases may be in remission or a quiescent phase, the need to fit in with peers can drive some nonadherence once they return to a more "normal" life. Creating a shared plan that takes into account the development stage of AYA and transitional patients and incorporates their individual values, beliefs, and goals can increase adherence to treatment and maintenance therapy. Palliative care providers are skilled at assessing patient's values, beliefs, and goals and translating those into plans (Carr & Rosengarten, 2021; Sansom-Daly, 2023; Pennarola et al., 2022).

2.6.5.2 Navigating Transitions

Transitions happen in myriad places and ways across health care settings (transition from inpatient to outpatient, transition from pediatric to adult care, transition to hospice, etc.). PPC providers are well positioned to help AYA patients navigate these transitions (Humphrey & Dell, 2015). For example, completing cancer-directed therapy and transitioning to survivorship is considered a good health care outcome; it can also be a time of emotional turmoil and loss for patients and families (Perez & Greenzang, 2019). Anxiety about no longer having regular visits and the support of the health care team often appears in patients and families during this time. Many patients feel things should go "back to normal" once treatment is complete, and others may have palliative care needs that extend beyond active treatment (Johnston & Rosenberg, 2023). Adjusting to the fact that there is a "new normal" requires normalization, and often validation, of frustrations and other emotions (Abdelhadi et al., 2022). Fear of recurrence can naturally lead to hypervigilance of symptoms and warrants a compassionate and clinically thorough approach to adequately evaluate concerns and provide guidance (Pulewka et al., 2021). The multidisciplinary team approach common in PPC can provide much of this support (Perez & Greenzang, 2019).

In the transition from pediatric to adult health care settings, PPC providers can facilitate communication among various team members and advocate for the patient.

During this transition, it is important to understand the patient's communication preferences around their illness as well as the type of information they need and wish to receive. For instance, transitional patients report an overwhelming need for more information on their disease and how to live healthily with it (Allen et al., 2022). PPC providers are skilled at identifying information, communication, and quality-of-life preferences and communicating those preferences to new providers (Frawley & Hebert, 2019; Allen et al., 2022). More research is needed to further delineate the role PPC plays in transitions as most studies focus on disease-specific transitions rather than need-based transitions (Doug et al., 2011).

2.6.5.3 Goal Establishment and Concordance

For adolescents and young adults with cancer and other serious illnesses, one thing they identify as most important is communication about their disease. Adolescents' abilities to engage meaningfully in these conversations vary widely, not just based on age. While some children as young as 8 years old can understand the meaning of death and can engage in discussions about dying, other patients and families may not be as open or as able to engage meaningfully (Longbottom & Slaughter, 2018). Adolescents and young adults can have difficulty articulating these new and strange feelings, consequently putting the onus on providers to identify these issues and bring them to light (Perez & Greenzang, 2019). PPC clinicians and team members, especially when involved early, can establish trusting relationships, leading to more goals of care conversations and more advance care planning (Sansom-Daly, 2023; Pennarola et al., 2022). Patients often report improved anxiety and less distress surrounding their diagnosis once they have had a chance to discuss these "taboo" subjects (Perez et al., 2020). PPC involvement offers the opportunity and a safe, guided place to have these discussions (Cavallo, 2021).

Providers' goals and patients' goals are not always aligned. To adolescents and young adults, other needs may take precedence over their health care (Smith et al., 2020). Some providers may assume the AYA or transitional patient's main goal is to prolong life; however, the goal of an AYA patient may be to just be normal—to make that movie night with their friends, or to go on that school trip. This may be seen by providers as the patient being "difficult" or shortsighted, even though it can be developmentally appropriate for AYA patients (McGrady & Pai, 2019; Darabos et al., 2023).

It is also important for providers to understand family-related goals an adolescent or AYA might have and respect them as family dynamic remains an especially important part of decisional support in this developmental stage. Serious illness affects not just the adolescent, but also families and caregivers. Many AYA patients report guilt for the family experiencing distress, both emotional and financial. Some may feel it is their fault and try anything they can to minimize family distress. Sometimes, this leads to being more passive in treatment, not wanting to "rock the boat," and going along with what their family or medical providers want to do (Straehla et al., 2017; Perez & Greenzang, 2019). This can be seen in particular when it comes to the location of death. One study showed that while most (67%) AYA patients preferred to die at home, many ended up dying in the hospital. There are assorted reasons for that, including not wanting to traumatize other family members (especially siblings), lack of home support/caregiving to meet the needs of the patient, and wanting to avoid placing strain on caregivers including parents or young spouses (Odejide et al., 2022). Additionally, while most patients prefer to be at home when they pass, most AYA patients also want to receive aggressive, life-prolonging care. When this leads to in-hospital deaths in older adults, it is often perceived as poor end-of-life quality and can lead to moral distress among staff; however, in an AYA patient, it may mean they received the best, most goal-concordant care (Ananth, 2021; Mack et al., 2021). Skilled communication by the PPC multidisciplinary team can help patients and families walk this fine line up through death and into bereavement. (Sanders et al., 2018; Sansom-Daly, 2023; Perez et al., 2020). PPC providers are also often needed to help staff reconcile the patient's expressed wish to die at home with the outcome of potentially dying in the hospital. However, this sort of reconciliation is only possible if discussions leading up to death are skilled and thorough, as noted above.

2.6.6 Specific Tools and Guidance for Addressing Particular Areas of Difficulty for AYA Patients

Various interventions have been found to improve quality of life and treatment adherence for adolescents and young adults. Online peer support groups, interactive apps, and/or medical devices (like an electronic water bottle to monitor fluid intake in end-stage renal disease) have all been used successfully. There may be promising hope in a video approach to discussing the basics of advanced care planning (Snaman et al., 2023). One-on-one counseling is more effective than large groups, and incorporating this principle in the multidisciplinary PPC team may help achieve greater psychological support (Pulewka et al., 2021).

Asking about joys, fears, and worries is one straightforward way to assess psychological and social needs for AYA and transitional patients; normalizing statements when addressing issues is another. Simply asking, "Some people experience x when going through y. Is that something you're experiencing or feeling right now?" can be a nonjudgmental way of exploring an adolescent or young adult's feelings (Perez & Greenzang, 2019). Normalize and provide reassurance that emotional responses to and coping with a serious illness are on a spectrum and that there is no "right way" to feel (Perez & Greenzang, 2019). Bringing these feelings up with family present can be a useful tool to facilitate communication between patients and families/caregivers, where each side can often hold in emotions to protect their loved ones. PPC providers can consider which approach to use with which patients and have the time to explore these issues.

Sexuality should also be approached as a normalized topic. Addressing hormone and/or fertility concerns can be a natural segue into the topic. Some AYA patients may appreciate a bit of humor with the approach. Most patients feel it is more likely to be addressed if brought up by the provider, rather than leaving it up to the patient to broach the subject (Albers et al., 2022). Given that adolescents with chronic illness are as likely (or more likely) to engage in risky behaviors (sexual, drug-related, etc.), they should undergo the same screening and anticipatory guidance (including sexual health topics) all adolescents receive (Albers et al., 2022; Suris & Parera, 2005).

A useful tool for advance care planning and goals of care discussions is the workbook Voicing My Choices, available through the Five Wishes website (https://www.fivewishes.org) (Zadeh et al., 2015). For those caring for AYA patients in survivorship, the Children's Oncology Group Long-Term Follow-up Guidelines (http://www.survivorshipguidelines.org/) are a great resource (Johnston & Rosenberg, 2023). For adolescents and young adults with chronic and other serious illness, Got Transitions (https://www.gottransition.org/) is a resource center on transitioning from pediatric to adult care.

2.6.7 Conclusion

Transitional and AYA patients can have suboptimal health care outcomes in the setting of their unique challenges. Particular care should be taken to evaluate each of these adolescents and young adults as individuals with distinct needs rather than a homogeneous group. Patients may be in various stages of development, and it is important for providers to meet them where they are. By approaching each new patient encounter with open-mindedness and curiosity, working with this population can be extremely rewarding. Many adolescents report positive experiences that come out of a serious illness, and it is a privilege to care for them as they navigate a time of challenge and change (Straehla et al., 2017; Greenzang et al., 2020).

References

Abdelhadi, O. A., Pollock, B. H., Joseph, J. G., & Keegan, T. H. M. (2022). Psychological distress and associated additional medical expenditures in adolescent and young adult cancer survivors. *Cancer, 128*(7), 1523–1531. https://doi.org/10.1002/cncr.34064

Afonso, N. S., Ninemire, M. R., Gowda, S. H., Jump, J. L., Lantin-Hermoso, R. L., Johnson, K. E., et al. (2021). Redefining the relationship: Palliative care in critical perinatal and neonatal cardiac patients. *Children (Basel), 8*(7), 548. https://doi.org/10.3390/children8070548

Albers, L. F., Bergsma, F. B., Mekelenkamp, H., Pelger, R. C. M., Manten-Horst, E., & Elzevier, H. W. (2022). Discussing sexual health with adolescent and young adults with cancer: A qualitative study among healthcare providers. *Journal of Cancer Education, 37*(1), 133–140. https://doi.org/10.1007/s13187-020-01796-0

Allen, T., Reda, S., Martin, S., Long, P., Franklin, A., Bedoya, S. Z., et al. (2022). The needs of adolescents and young adults with chronic illness: Results of a quality improvement survey. *Children (Basel), 9*(4), 500. https://doi.org/10.3390/children9040500

American Academy of Pediatrics (AAP) Committee on Children with Disabilities and Committee on Psychosocial Aspects of Child and Family Health. (1993). Psychosocial risks of chronic health conditions in childhood and adolescence. *Pediatrics, 92*(6), 876–878. https://doi.org/10.1542/peds.92.6.876

American Academy of Pediatrics (AAP) Committee on Bioethics and Committee on Hospital Care. (2000). Palliative care for children. *Pediatrics, 106*(2), 351–357. https://doi.org/10.1542/peds.106.2.351

American College of Obstetricians and Gynecologists (ACOG). (2019). Perinatal palliative care: ACOG committee opinion number 786. *Obstetrics & Gynecology, 134*(3), e84–e89. https://doi.org/10.1097/AOG.0000000000003425

Ananth, P. (2021). Reenvisioning end-of-life care quality measurement for adolescents and young adults with cancer-novel patient-centered indicators and approaches. *JAMA Network Open, 4*(8), e2122323. https://doi.org/10.1001/jamanetworkopen.2021.22323

Baker, J. N., Torkildson, C., Baillargeon, J. G., Olney, C. A., & Kane, J. R. (2007). National survey of pediatric residency program directors and residents regarding education in palliative medicine and end-of-life care. *Journal of Palliative Medicine, 10*(2), 420–429. https://doi.org/10.1089/jpm.2006.0135

Baker, J. N., Hinds, P. S., Spunt, S. L., Barfield, R. C., Allen, C., Powell, B. C., Anderson, L. H., & Kane, J. R. (2008). Integration of palliative care practices into the ongoing care of children with cancer: Individualized care planning and coordination. *Pediatric Clinics of North America, 55*(1), 223–250. https://doi.org/10.1016/j.pcl.2007.10.011

Balkin, E. M., Kirkpatrick, J. N., Kaufman, B., Swetz, K. M., Sleeper, L. A., Wolfe, J., et al. (2017). Pediatric cardiology provider attitudes about palliative care: A multicenter survey study. *Pediatric Cardiology, 38*(7), 1324–1331. https://doi.org/10.1007/s00246-017-1663-0

Bellizzi, K. M., Smith, A., Schmidt, S., Keegan, T. H., Zebrack, B., Lynch, C. F., Deapen, D., Shnorhavorian, M., Tompkins, B. J., & Simon, M. (2012). Positive and negative psychosocial impact of being diagnosed with cancer as an adolescent or young adult. *Cancer, 118*(20), 5155–5162. https://doi.org/10.1002/cncr.27512

Bergsträsser, E., Lukose, S., Zimmermann, K., & Oxenius, A. (2022). Palliative care in children with advanced heart disease in a tertiary care environment: A mini review. *Frontiers in Cardiovascular Medicine, 9*, 863031. https://doi.org/10.3389/fcvm.2022.863031

Blume, E. D., Kirsch, R., Cousino, M. K., Walter, J. K., Steiner, J. M., Miller, T. A., Machado, D., Peyton, C., Bacha, E., Morell, E., & American Heart Association Pediatric Heart Failure and Transplantation Committee of the Council on Lifelong Congenital Heart Disease and Heart Health in the Young (2023). Palliative Care Across the Life Span for Children With Heart Disease: A Scientific Statement From the American Heart Association. Circulation. Cardiovascular quality and outcomes, 16(2), e000114. https://doi.org/10.1161/HCQ.0000000000000114

Boan Pion, A., Baenziger, J., Fauchère, J. C., Gubler, D., & Hendriks, M. J. (2021). National divergences in perinatal palliative care guidelines and training in tertiary NICUs. *Frontiers in Pediatrics, 9*, 673545. https://doi.org/10.3389/fped.2021.673545

Bogetz, J. F., Ullrich, C. K., & Berry, J. G. (2014). Pediatric hospital care for children with life-threatening illness and the role of palliative care. *Pediatric Clinics of North America, 61*(4), 719–733.

Bogetz, J. F., Trowbridge, A., Lewis, H., Shipman, K. J., Jonas, D., Hauer, J., & Rosenberg, A. R. (2021). Parents are the experts: A qualitative study of the experiences of parents of children with severe neurological impairment during decision-making. *Journal of Pain and Symptom Management, 62*(6), 1117–1125. https://doi.org/10.1016/j.jpainsymman.2021.06.011

Borasio, G. D. (2013). The role of palliative care in patients with neurological diseases. *Nature Reviews Neurology, 9*(5), 292–295. https://doi.org/10.1038/nrneurol.2013.49

Boss, R., Nelson, J., Weissman, D., Campbell, M., Curtis, R., Frontera, J., Gabriel, M., Lustbader, D., Mosenthal, A., & Mulkerin, C. (2014). Integrating palliative care into the PICU: A report from the improving palliative care in the ICU Advisory Board. *Pediatric Critical Care Medicine, 15*(8), 762–7677. https://doi.org/10.1097/PCC.0000000000000209

Carr, E., & Rosengarten, L. (2021). Teenagers and young adults with cancer: An exploration of factors contributing to treatment adherence. *Journal of Pediatric Oncology Nursing, 38*(3), 190–204. https://doi.org/10.1177/1043454221992302

Cavallo, J. (2021, June 25). How to talk with teens and young adults about their end-of-life goals. *The ASCO Post.* https://ascopost.com/issues/june-25-2021/how-to-talk-with-teens-and-young-adults-about-their-end-of-life-goals/

Center to Advance Palliative Care (CAPC). (2022, March 2). *Pediatric palliative care referral criteria.* Retrieved March 18, 2024, from https://www.capc.org/documents/288/

Cheng, B. T., & Wangmo, T. (2020). Palliative care utilization in hospitalized children with cancer. *Pediatric Blood & Cancer, 67*(1), e28013. https://doi.org/10.1002/pbc.28013

Ciriello, A. G., Dizon, Z. B., October, T. W. (2018). Speaking a Different Language: A Qualitative Analysis Comparing Language of Palliative Care and Pediatric Intensive Care Unit Physicians. *American Journal of Hospice and Palliative Medicine, 35*(3):384–389. https://doi.org/10.1177/1049909117700101

Cohen, E., Kuo, D. Z., Agrawal, R., Berry, J. G., Bhagat, S. K., Simon, T. D., & Srivastava, R. (2011). Children with medical complexity: An emerging population for clinical and research initiatives. *Pediatrics, 127*(3), 529–538. https://doi.org/10.1542/peds.2010-0910

Contro, N., Larson, J., Scofield, S., Sourkes, B., & Cohen, H. (2002). Family perspectives on the quality of pediatric palliative care. *Archives of Pediatrics & Adolescent Medicine, 156*(1), 14–19. https://doi.org/10.1001/archpedi.156.1.14

Cortezzo, D. E., Ellis, K., & Schlegel, A. (2020). Perinatal palliative care birth planning as advance care planning. *Frontiers in Pediatrics, 8*, 556. https://doi.org/10.3389/fped.2020.00556

Dalberg, T., Jacob-Files, E., Carney, P. A., Meyrowitz, J., Fromme, E. K., & Thomas, G. (2013). Pediatric oncology providers' perceptions of barriers and facilitators to early integration of pediatric palliative care. *Pediatric Blood & Cancer, 60*(11), 1875–1881. https://doi.org/10.1002/pbc.24673

Dallara, A., Meret, A., & Saroyan, J. (2014). Mapping the literature: Palliative care within adult and child neurology. *Journal of Child Neurology, 29*(12), 1728–1738. https://doi.org/10.1177/0883073814527159

Darabos, K., Tucker, C. A., Brumley, L., King-Dowling, S., Butler, E., Stevens, E., O'Hagan, B., Henry-Moss, D., Deatrick, J. A., Szala, D., Barakat, L. P., & Schwartz, L. A. (2023). Development and validation of a measure of adolescent and young adult goal-based quality of life (MAYA-GQOL). *Quality of Life Research, 32*(8), 2305–2317. https://doi.org/10.1007/s11136-023-03392-3

Davis, A. M., McFadden, S. E., Patterson, B. L., & Barkin, S. L. (2015). Strategies to identify and stratify children with special health care needs in outpatient general pediatrics settings. *Maternal and Child Health Journal, 19*(6), 1384–1392. https://doi.org/10.1007/s10995-014-1644-3

Defanti, C. A., & Ad Hoc Working Group of the Italian Neurological Society. (2000). Study Group of Bioethics and Palliative Care in Neurology: Program document. *Neurological Sciences, 21*(5), 261–271. https://doi.org/10.1007/s100720070062

Delgado-Corcoran, C., Wawrzynski, S. E., Bennett, E. E., Green, D., Bodily, S., Moore, D., Cook, L. J., & Olson, L. M. (2020). Palliative care in children with heart disease treated in an ICU. *Pediatric Critical Care Medicine, 21*(5), 423–429. https://doi.org/10.1097/PCC.0000000000002271

Dombrecht, L., Chambaere, K., Beernaert, K., Roets, E., De Vilder De Keyser, M., De Smet, G., Roelens, K., & Cools, F. (2023). Components of perinatal palliative care: An integrative review. *Children (Basel), 10*(3), 482. https://doi.org/10.3390/children10030482

Doug, M., Adi, Y., Williams, J., Paul, M., Kelly, D., Petchey, R., & Carter, Y. H. (2011). Transition to adult services for children and young people with palliative care needs: A systematic review. *Archives of Disease in Childhood, 96*(1), 78–84. https://doi.org/10.1136/adc.2009.163931

El-Jawahri, A., Greer, J. A., Pirl, W. F., Park, E. R., Jackson, V. A., Back, A. L., Kamdar, M., Jacobsen, J., Chittenden, E. H., Rinaldi, S. P., Gallagher, E. R., Eusebio, J. R., Fishman, S., VanDusen, H., Li, Z., Muzikansky, A., & Temel, J. S. (2017). Effects of early integrated palliative care on caregivers of patients with lung and gastrointestinal cancer: A randomized clinical trial. *The Oncologist, 22*(12), 1528–1534. https://doi.org/10.1634/theoncologist.2017-0227

English, N. K., & Hessler, K. L. (2013). Prenatal birth planning for families of the imperiled newborn. *Journal of Obstetric, Gynecologic, & Neonatal Nursing, 42*(3), 390–399. https://doi.org/10.1111/1552-6909.12031

Ferrari, A., Stark, D., Peccatori, F. A., Fern, L., Laurence, V., Gaspar, N., Bozovic-Spasojevic, I., Smith, O., De Munter, J., Derwich, K., Hjorth, L., van der Graaf, W. T. A., Soanes, L., Jezdic, S., Blondeel, A., Bielack, S., Douillard, J. Y., Mountzios, G., & Saloustros, E. (2021). Adolescents and young adults (AYA) with cancer: A position paper from the AYA working Group of the European Society for Medical Oncology (ESMO) and the European Society for Paediatric Oncology (SIOPE). *ESMO Open, 6*(2), 100096. https://doi.org/10.1016/j.esmoop.2021.100096

Ferrell, B. R., Temel, J. S., Temin, S., Alesi, E. R., Balboni, T. A., Basch, E. M., Firn, J. I., Paice, J. A., Peppercorn, J. M., Phillips, T., Stovall, E. L., Zimmermann, C., & Smith, T. J. (2017). Integration of palliative care into standard oncology care: American Society of Clinical Oncology clinical practice guideline update. *Journal of Clinical Oncology, 35*(1), 96–112. https://doi.org/10.1200/JCO.2016.70.1474

Ferrell, B. R., Twaddle, M. L., Melnick, A., & Meier, D. E. (2018). National consensus project clinical practice guidelines for quality palliative care guidelines, 4th edition. *Journal of Palliative Medicine, 21*(12), 1684–1689. https://doi.org/10.1089/jpm.2018.0431

Feudtner, C., Kang, T. I., Hexem, K. R., Friedrichsdorf, S. J., Osenga, K., Siden, H., Friebert, S. E., Hays, R. M., Dussel, V., & Wolfe, J. (2011). Pediatric palliative care patients: A prospective multicenter cohort study. *Pediatrics, 127*(6), 1094–1101. https://doi.org/10.1542/peds.2010-3225

Fraser, L. K., van Laar, M., Miller, M., Aldridge, J., McKinney, P. A., Parslow, R. C., & Feltbower, R. (2013). Does referral to specialist paediatric palliative care services reduce hospital admissions in oncology patients at the end of life? *British Journal of Cancer, 108*(6), 1273–1279. https://doi.org/10.1038/bjc.2013.89

Frawley, J., & Hebert, R. (2019, March 6). *Fast fact #346: Seriously ill pediatric patients who transition to adulthood*. Palliative Care Network of Wisconsin. Retrieved February 2, 2024, from https://www.mypcnow.org/fast-fact/seriously-ill-pediatric-patients-who-transition-to-adulthood/

Friebert S, & Osenga K. (2022, March 2). *Pediatric palliative care referral criteria*. Center to Advance Palliative Care. Retrieved January 24, 2024, from https://www.capc.org/toolkits/

Friedrichsdorf, S. J., Postier, A., Dreyfus, J., Osenga, K., Sencer, S., & Wolfe, J. (2015). Improved quality of life at end of life related to home-based palliative care in children with cancer. *Journal of Palliative Medicine, 18*(2), 143–150. https://doi.org/10.1089/jpm.2014.0285

Ghandour, R. M., Hirai, A. H., & Kenney, M. K. (2022). Children and youth with special health care needs: A profile. *Pediatrics, 149*(Suppl 7), e2021056150D. https://doi.org/10.1542/peds.2021-056150D

Gilboa, S. M., Devine, O. J., Kucik, J. E., Oster, M. E., Riehle-Colarusso, T., Nembhard, W. N., Xu, P., Correa, A., Jenkins, K., & Marelli, A. J. (2016). Congenital heart defects in the United States: Estimating the magnitude of the affected population in 2010. *Circulation, 134*(2), 101–109. https://doi.org/10.1161/CIRCULATIONAHA.115.019307

Goloff, N., & Joy, B. F. (2018). A part of the team: The changing role of palliative care in congenital heart disease. *Progress in Pediatric Cardiology, 48*, 59–62. https://doi.org/10.1016/j.ppedcard.2018.01.009

Graaf, G., & Gigli, K. (2022). Care coordination and unmet need for specialised health services among children with special healthcare needs in the USA: Results from a cross-sectional analysis of the national survey of children with special healthcare needs. *BMJ Open, 12*(11), e063373. https://doi.org/10.1136/bmjopen-2022-063373

Green, D. J., Bennett, E., Olson, L. M., Wawrzynski, S., Bodily, S., Moore, D., Mansfield, K. J., Wilkins, V., Cook, L., & Delgado-Corcoran, C. (2021). Timing of pediatric palliative care consults in hospitalized patients with heart disease. *Journal of Pediatric Intensive Care, 12*(1), 63–67. https://doi.org/10.1055/s-0041-1730916

Greenzang, K. A., Fasciano, K. M., Block, S. D., & Mack, J. W. (2020). Early information needs of adolescents and young adults about late effects of cancer treatment. *Cancer, 126*(14), 3281–3288. https://doi.org/10.1002/cncr.32932

Haines, E. R., Frost, A. C., Kane, H. L., & Rokoske, F. S. (2018). Barriers to accessing palliative care for pediatric patients with cancer: A review of the literature. *Cancer, 124*(11), 2278–2288. https://doi.org/10.1002/cncr.31265

Hancock, H. S., Pituch, K., Uzark, K., Bhat, P., Fifer, C., Silveira, M., Sunkyung, Y., Welch, S., Donohue, J., Lowery, R., & Aiyagari, R. (2018). A randomised trial of early palliative care for maternal stress in infants prenatally diagnosed with single-ventricle heart disease. *Cardiology in the Young, 28*(4), 561–570. https://doi.org/10.1017/S1047951117002761

Hauer, J. M., & Wolfe, J. (2014). Supportive and palliative care of children with metabolic and neurological diseases. *Current Opinion in Supportive and Palliative Care, 8*(3), 296–302. https://doi.org/10.1097/SPC.0000000000000063

Headrick, A., Wawrzynski, S. E., De Leon Jauregui, M., Moore, J., Winder, M. M., Moresco, B., Moore, D., Millar, M. M., Codden, R., & Delgado-Corcoran, C. (2023, October 20–24). *A discrete trigger to increase specialized palliative care consultation in children with heart disease and prolonged cardiac intensive care unit hospitalization: A quality improvement project* [Poster Abstract]. 2023 AAP national conference and exhibition, Washington, DC, USA. https://aapexperience23.eventscribe.net/aaStatic.asp?SFP=RIlORINNWURAMTYzNzk

Health Resources and Services Administration Maternal and Child Health Bureau (MCHB). (2022). *National survey of children's health: Children and youth with special health care needs data brief.* https://mchb.hrsa.gov/data-research/national-survey-childrens-health.

Hepgul, N., Gao, W., Evans, C. J., Jackson, D., van Vliet, L. M., Byrne, A., Crosby, V., Groves, K. E., Lindsay, F., Higginson, I. J., & OPTCARE Neuro. (2018). Integrating palliative care into neurology services: What do the professionals say? *BMJ Supportive & Palliative Care, 8*(1), 41–44.

Hilden, J. (2016). It is time to let in pediatric palliative care. *Pediatric Blood & Cancer, 63*(4), 583–584. https://doi.org/10.1002/pbc.25877

Ho, C., & Straatman, L. (2013). A review of pediatric palliative care service utilization in children with a progressive neuromuscular disease who died on a palliative care program. *Journal of Child Neurology, 28*(1), 40–44. https://doi.org/10.1177/0883073812439345

Hoegy, D., Guilloux, R., Bleyzac, N., Gauthier-Vasserot, A., Cannas, G., Bertrand, Y., Dussart, C., & Janoly-Dumenil, A. (2022). Pediatric-adult care transition: Perceptions of adolescent and young adult patients with sickle cell disease and their healthcare providers. *Patient Preference and Adherence, 16*, 2727–2737. https://doi.org/10.2147/PPA.S377236

Houtrow, A., Martin, A. J., Harris, D., Cejas, D., Hutson, R., Mazloomdoost, Y., & Agrawal, R. K. (2022). Health equity for children and youth with special health care needs: A vision for the future. *Pediatrics, 149*(Suppl 7), e2021056150F. https://doi.org/10.1542/peds.2021-056150F

Humphrey, L., & Dell, M. L. (2015). Identifying the unique aspects of adolescent and young adult palliative care: A case study to propel programmatic changes in pediatric hospitals. *Seminars in Pediatric Neurology, 22*(3), 166–171. https://doi.org/10.1016/j.spen.2015.05.006

Humphrey, L., & Kang, T. I. (2015). Palliative care in pediatric patients with hematologic malignancies. *Hematology. American Society of Hematology. Education Program, 2015*, 490–495. https://doi.org/10.1182/asheducation-2015.1.490

Jarvis, S. W., Roberts, D., Flemming, K., Richardson, G., & Fraser, L. K. (2021). Transition of children with life-limiting conditions to adult care and healthcare use: A systematic review. *Pediatric Research, 90*(6), 1120–1131. https://doi.org/10.1038/s41390-021-01396-8

Jetha, M., & Segalowitz, S. (2012). *Adolescent brain development.* Academic Press.

Johnston, E. E., & Rosenberg, A. R. (2023). Palliative care in adolescents and young adults with cancer. *Journal of Clinical Oncology, 42*(6), 755–763. https://doi.org/10.1200/jco.23.00709

Kassam, A., Skiadaresis, J., Alexander, S., & Wolfe, J. (2015). Differences in end-of-life communication for children with advanced cancer who were referred to a palliative care team. *Pediatric Blood & Cancer, 62*(8), 1409–1413. https://doi.org/10.1002/pbc.25530

Kaye, E. C., Friebert, S., & Baker, J. N. (2016). Early integration of palliative care for children with high-risk cancer and their families. *Pediatric Blood & Cancer, 63*(4), 593–597. https://doi.org/10.1002/pbc.25848

Kaye, E. C., Kiefer, A., Blazin, L., Spraker-Perlman, H., Clark, L., & Baker, J. N. (2020). Bereaved parents, hope, and realism. *Pediatrics, 145*(5), e20192771. https://doi.org/10.1542/peds.2019-2771

Kaye, E. C., Rockwell, S., Woods, C., Lemmon, M. E., Andes, K., Baker, J. N., & Mack, J. W. (2021a). Facilitators associated with building and sustaining therapeutic alliance in advanced pediatric cancer. *JAMA Network Open, 4*(8), e2120925. https://doi.org/10.1001/jamanetworkopen.2021.20925

Kaye, E. C., Weaver, M. S., DeWitt, L. H., Byers, E., Stevens, S. E., Lukowski, J., Shih, B., Zalud, K., Applegarth, J., Wong, H. N., Baker, J. N., Ullrich, C. K., & AAHPM Research Committee. (2021b). The impact of specialty palliative care in pediatric oncology: A systematic review. *Journal of Pain and Symptom Management, 61*(5), 1060–1079.e2. https://doi.org/10.1016/j.jpainsymman.2020.12.003

Kaye, E. C., Woods, C., Kennedy, K., Velrajan, S., Gattas, M., Bilbeisi, T., Huber, R., Lemmon, M. E., Baker, J. N., & Mack, J. W. (2021c). Communication around palliative care principles and advance care planning between oncologists, children with advancing cancer and families. *British Journal of Cancer, 125*(8), 1089–1099. https://doi.org/10.1038/s41416-021-01512-9

Keim-Malpass, J., Hart, T. G., & Miller, J. R. (2013). Coverage of palliative and hospice care for pediatric patients with a life-limiting illness: A policy brief. *Journal of Pediatric Health Care, 27*(6), 511–516. https://doi.org/10.1016/j.pedhc.2013.07.011

Kirchhoff, A. C., Fowler, B., Warner, E. L., Pannier, S. T., Fair, D., Spraker-Perlman, H., Yancey, J., Bott, B., Reynolds, C., & Randall, R. L. (2017). Supporting adolescents and young adults with cancer: Oncology provider perceptions of adolescent and young adult unmet needs. *Journal of Adolescent and Young Adult Oncology, 6*(4), 519–523. https://doi.org/10.1089/jayao.2017.0011

Klijn, N. F., Ter Kuile, M. M., & Lashley, E. E. L. O. (2023). Patient-reported outcomes (PROs) and patient experiences in fertility preservation: A systematic review of the literature on adolescents and young adults (AYAs) with cancer. *Cancers (Basel), 15*(24), 5828. https://doi.org/10.3390/cancers15245828

Kumar, M. M. (2023). Eating disorders in youth with chronic health conditions: Clinical strategies for early recognition and prevention. *Nutrients, 15*(17), 3672. https://doi.org/10.3390/nu15173672

Kuo, D. Z., Houtrow, A. J., & Council on Children with Disabilities. (2016). Recognition and management of medical complexity. *Pediatrics, 138*(6), e20163021. https://doi.org/10.1542/peds.2016-3021

Levine, D. R., Mandrell, B. N., Sykes, A., Pritchard, M., Gibson, D., Symons, H. J., Wendler, D., & Baker, J. N. (2017). Patients' and parents' needs, attitudes, and perceptions about early palliative care integration in pediatric oncology. *JAMA Oncology, 3*(9), 1214–1220. https://doi.org/10.1001/jamaoncol.2017.0368

Lo, D. S., Hein, N., & Bulgareli, J. V. (2022). Pediatric palliative care and end-of-life: A systematic review of economic health analyses. *Revista Paulista de Pediatria, 40*, e2021002. https://doi.org/10.1590/1984-0462/2022/40/2021002

Longbottom, S., & Slaughter, V. (2018). Sources of children's knowledge about death and dying. *Philosophical Transactions of the Royal Society of London Series B, Biological Sciences, 373*(1754), 20170267. https://doi.org/10.1098/rstb.2017.0267

Lowenstein, S., Macauley, R., Perko, K., & Ronai, C. (2020). Provider perspective on the role of palliative care in hypoplastic left heart syndrome. *Cardiology in the Young, 30*(3), 377–382. https://doi.org/10.1017/S1047951120000128

Lyons-Warren, A. M., Stowe, R. C., Emrick, L., & Jarrell, J. A. (2019). Early identification of pediatric neurology patients with palliative care needs: A pilot study. *American Journal of Hospice & Palliative Care, 36*(11), 959–966. https://doi.org/10.1177/1049909119844519

Mack, J. W., & Wolfe, J. (2006). Early integration of pediatric palliative care: For some children, palliative care starts at diagnosis. *Current Opinion in Pediatrics, 18*(1), 10–14. https://doi.org/10.1097/01.mop.0000193266.86129.47

Mack, J. W., Chen, L. H., Cannavale, K., Sattayapiwat, O., Cooper, R., & Chao, C. (2015). End-of-life care intensity among adolescent and young adult patients with cancer in Kaiser Permanente Southern California. *JAMA Oncology, 1*(5), 592. https://doi.org/10.1001/jamaoncol.2015.1953

Mack, J. W., Fisher, L., Kushi, L., Chao, C. R., Vega, B., Rodrigues, G., Joshephs, I., Brock, K. E., Buchanan, S., Casperson, M., Cooper, R. M., Fasciano, K. M., Kolevska, T., Lakin, J. R., Lefebvre, A., Schwartz, C. M., Shalman, D. M., Wall, C. B., Wiener, L., & Altschuler, A. (2021). Patient, family, and clinician perspectives on end-of-life care quality domains and candidate indicators for adolescents and young adults with cancer. *JAMA Network Open, 4*(8), e2121888. https://doi.org/10.1001/jamanetworkopen.2021.21888

Marcus, K. L., Balkin, E. M., Al-Sayegh, H., Guslits, E., Blume, E. D., Ma, C., & Wolfe, J. (2018). Patterns and outcomes of care in children with advanced heart disease receiving palliative care consultation. *Journal of Pain and Symptom Management, 55*(2), 351–358. https://doi.org/10.1016/j.jpainsymman.2017.08.033

McGrady, M. E., & Pai, A. L. H. (2019). A systematic review of rates, outcomes, and predictors of medication non-adherence among adolescents and young adults with cancer. *Journal of Adolescent and Young Adult Oncology, 8*(5), 485–494. https://doi.org/10.1089/jayao.2018.0160

Mitchell, S., Morris, A., Bennett, K., Sajid, L., & Dale, J. (2017). Specialist paediatric palliative care services: What are the benefits? *Archives of Disease in Childhood, 102*(10), 923–929. https://doi.org/10.1136/archdischild-2016-312026

Morell, E., Thompson, J., Rajagopal, S., Blume, E. D., & May, R. (2021). Congenital cardiothoracic surgeons and palliative care: A national survey study. *Journal of Palliative Care, 36*(1), 17–21. https://doi.org/10.1177/0825859719874765

Moynihan, K. M., Snaman, J. M., Kaye, E. C., Morrison, W. E., DeWitt, A. G., Sacks, L. D., Thompson, J. L., Hwang, J. M., Bailey, V., Lafond, D. A., Wolfe, J., & Blume, E. D. (2019). Integration of pediatric palliative care into cardiac intensive care: A champion-based model. *Pediatrics, 144*(2), e20190160. https://doi.org/10.1542/peds.2019-0160

Moynihan, K. M., Heith, C. S., Snaman, J. M., Smith-Parrish, M., Bakas, A., Ge, S., Cerqueira, A. V., Bailey, V., Beke, D., Wolfe, J., Morell, E., Gauvreau, K., & Blume, E. D. (2021). Palliative care referrals in cardiac disease. *Pediatrics, 147*(3), e2020018580. https://doi.org/10.1542/peds.2020-018580

National Cancer Institute. (2024, February 15). *Adolescents and young adults with cancer.* Retrieved February 29, 2024, from https://www.cancer.gov/types/aya

National Cancer Institute Division of Cancer Control & Population Sciences. (2023, November 30). *Patient-reported outcomes version of the common terminology criteria for adverse events (PRO-CTCAE®).* Retrieved February 29, 2024, from https://healthcaredelivery.cancer.gov/pro-ctcae/

National Hospice and Palliative Care Organization (NHPCO). (2022). *Standards of practice for pediatric palliative care.* Retrieved March 20, 2024, from https://www.nhpco.org/wp-content/uploads/Pediatric_Standards.pdf

Newman, H., & Hunger, S. P. (2023). Future of treatment of adolescents and young adults with ALL: A vision for collaboration and equity. *Journal of Clinical Oncology, 42*(6), 665–674. https://doi.org/10.1200/JCO.23.01351

Odejide, O. O., Fisher, L., Kushi, L. H., Chao, C., Vega, B., Rodrigues, G., Josephs, I., Brock, K. E., Buchanan, S., Casperson, M., Cooper, R., Fasciano, K., Kolevska, T., Lakin, J. R., Lefebvre, A., Schwartz, C. M., Shalman, D., Wall, C. B., Wiener, L., et al. (2022). Patient, family, and clinician perspectives on location of death for adolescents and young adults with cancer. *JCO Oncology Practice, 18*(10), e1621–e1629. https://doi.org/10.1200/op.22.00143

Olagunju, A. T., Sarimiye, F. O., Olagunju, T. O., Habeebu, M. Y., & Aina, O. F. (2016). Child's symptom burden and depressive symptoms among caregivers of children with cancers: An argument for early integration of pediatric palliative care. *Annals of Palliative Medicine, 5*(3), 157–165. https://doi.org/10.21037/apm.2016.04.03

Oliver, D. J., Borasio, G. D., Caraceni, A., de Visser, M., Grisold, W., Lorenzl, S., Veronese, S., & Voltz, R. (2016). A consensus review on the development of palliative care for patients with chronic and progressive neurological disease. *European Journal of Neurology, 23*(1), 30–38. https://doi.org/10.1111/ene.12889

Parsons, S. K., Keegan, T. H. M., Kirchhoff, A. C., Parsons, H. M., Yabroff, K. R., & Davies, S. J. (2023). Cost of cancer in adolescents and young adults in the United States: Results of the 2021 report by Deloitte Access Economics, commissioned by Teen Cancer America. *Journal of Clinical Oncology, 41*(17), 3260–3268. https://doi.org/10.1200/JCO.22.01985

Pennarola, B. W., Fry, A., Prichett, L., Beri, A. E., Shah, N. N., & Wiener, L. (2022). Mapping the landscape of advance care planning in adolescents and young adults receiving allogeneic hematopoietic stem cell transplantation: A 5-year retrospective review. *Transplantation and Cellular Therapy, 28*(3), 164.e1–164.e8. https://doi.org/10.1016/j.jtct.2021.12.007

Perez, S., & Greenzang, K. A. (2019). Completion of adolescent cancer treatment: Excitement, guilt, and anxiety. *Pediatrics, 143*(3), e20183073. https://doi.org/10.1542/peds.2018-3073

Perez, G. K., Salsman, J. M., Fladeboe, K., Kirchhoff, A. C., Park, E. R., & Rosenberg, A. R. (2020). Taboo topics in adolescent and young adult oncology: Strategies for managing challenging but important conversations central to adolescent and young adult cancer survivorship. *American Society of Clinical Oncology. Annual Meeting, 40*, 1–15. https://doi.org/10.1200/EDBK_279787

Provinciali, L., Carlini, G., Tarquini, D., Defanti, C. A., Veronese, S., & Pucci, E. (2016). Need for palliative care for neurological diseases. *Neurological Sciences, 37*(10), 1581–1587. https://doi.org/10.1007/s10072-016-2614-x

Pulewka, K., Strauss, B., Hochhaus, A., & Hilgendorf, I. (2021). Clinical, social, and psycho-oncological needs of adolescents and young adults (AYA) versus older patients following hematopoietic stem cell transplantation. *Journal of Cancer Research and Clinical Oncology, 147*(4), 1239–1246. https://doi.org/10.1007/s00432-020-03419-z

Reinman, L., Coons, H. L., Sopfe, J., & Casey, R. (2021). Psychosexual care of adolescent and young adult (AYA) cancer survivors. *Children (Basel), 8*(11), 1058. https://doi.org/10.3390/children8111058

Richards, C. A., Starks, H., O'Connor, M. R., Bourget, E., Lindhorst, T., Hays, R., & Doorenbos, A. Z. (2018). When and why do neonatal and pediatric critical care physicians consult palliative care? *American Journal of Hospice & Palliative Care, 35*(6), 840–846. https://doi.org/10.1177/1049909117739853

Roman, S. B., Dworkin, P. H., Dickinson, P., & Rogers, S. C. (2020). Analysis of care coordination needs for families of children with special health care needs. *Journal of Developmental & Behavioral Pediatrics, 41*(1), 58–64. https://doi.org/10.1097/DBP.0000000000000734

Sanders, J., Curtis, J. R., & Tulsky, J. A. (2018). Achieving goal-concordant care: A conceptual model and approach to measuring serious illness communication and its impact. *Journal of Palliative Medicine, 21*(S2), S17–S27. https://doi.org/10.1089/jpm.2017.0459

Sansom-Daly, U. M. (2023). Specialty palliative care for adolescents and young adults with cancer-developmental considerations and an agenda for future research. *JAMA Network Open, 6*(10), e2338681. https://doi.org/10.1001/jamanetworkopen.2023.38681

Schiff, J., Manning, L., VanLandeghem, K., Langer, C. S., Schutze, M., & Comeau, M. (2022). Financing care for CYSHCN in the next decade: Reducing burden, advancing equity, and transforming systems. *Pediatrics, 149*(Suppl 7), e2021056150I. https://doi.org/10.1542/peds.2021-056150I

Schmidt, P., Otto, M., Hechler, T., Metzing, S., Wolfe, J., & Zernikow, B. (2013). Did increased availability of pediatric palliative care lead to improved palliative care outcomes in children with cancer? *Journal of Palliative Medicine, 16*(9), 1034–1039. https://doi.org/10.1089/jpm.2013.0014

Shnorhavorian, M., Harlan, L. C., Smith, A. W., Keegan, T. H., Lynch, C. F., Prasad, P. K., Cress, R. D., Wu, X. C., Hamilton, A. S., Parsons, H. M., Keel, G., Charlesworth, S. E., Schwartz, S. M., & AYA HOPE Study Collaborative Group. (2015). Fertility preservation knowledge, counseling, and actions among adolescent and young adult patients with cancer: A population-based study. *Cancer, 121*(19), 3499–3506. https://doi.org/10.1002/cncr.29328

Siegel, D. A., King, J. B., Lupo, P. J., Durbin, E. B., Tai, E., Mills, K., Van Dyne, E., Buchanan Lunsford, N., Henley, S. J., & Wilson, R. J. (2023a). Counts, incidence rates, and trends of pediatric cancer in the United States, 2003–2019. *Journal of the National Cancer Institute, 115*(11), 1337–1354. https://doi.org/10.1093/jnci/djad115

Siegel, R. L., Miller, K. D., Wagle, N. S., & Jemal, A. (2023b). Cancer statistics, 2023. *CA: A Cancer Journal for Clinicians, 73*(1), 17–48. https://doi.org/10.3322/caac.21763

Smith, A. W., Keegan, T. H., Hamilton, A. S., Lynch, C. F., Wu, X., Schwartz, S. M., Kato, I., Cress, R. D., & Harlan, L. C. (2018). Understanding care and outcomes in adolescents and young adults with cancer: A review of the AYA HOPE study. *Pediatric Blood & Cancer, 66*(1), e27486. https://doi.org/10.1002/pbc.27486

Smith, L., Critoph, D. J., & Hatcher, H. (2020). How can health care professionals communicate effectively with adolescent and young adults who have completed cancer treatment? A systematic review. *Journal of Adolescent and Young Adult Oncology, 9*(3), 328–340. https://doi.org/10.1089/jayao.2019.0133

Snaman, J. M., Kaye, E. C., Lu, J. J., Sykes, A., & Baker, J. N. (2017). Palliative care involvement is associated with less intensive end-of-life care in adolescent and young adult oncology patients. *Journal of Palliative Medicine, 20*(5), 509–516. https://doi.org/10.1089/jpm.2016.0451

Snaman, J. M., Talleur, A. C., Lu, J., Levine, D. R., Kaye, E. C., Sykes, A., Lu, Z., Triplett, B. M., & Baker, J. N. (2018). Treatment intensity and symptom burden in hospitalized adolescent and young adult hematopoietic cell transplant recipients at the end of life. *Bone Marrow Transplantation, 53*(1), 84–90. https://doi.org/10.1038/bmt.2017.187

Snaman, J., McCarthy, S., Wiener, L., & Wolfe, J. (2020). Pediatric palliative care in oncology. *Journal of Clinical Oncology, 38*(9), 954–962. https://doi.org/10.1200/JCO.18.02331

Snaman, J. M., Feifer, D., Helton, G., Chang, Y., El-Jawahri, A., Volandes, A. E., & Wolfe, J. (2023). A pilot randomized trial of an advance care planning video decision support tool for adolescents and young adults with advanced cancer. *Journal of the National Comprehensive Cancer Network, 21*(7), 715–723.e17. https://doi.org/10.6004/jnccn.2023.7021

Songer, K., Wawrzynski, S. E., Olson, L., & Delgado-Corcoran, C. (2023, August 27–September 1). *Effect of timing of palliative care consultation on end-of-life care for children with advanced cardiac disease.* [Poster presentation]. 8th World congress of pediatric cardiology and cardiac surgery, Washington, DC, USA. https://www.wcpccs2023.org/event/1da8563e-0f65-486c-88df-70c3db431af5/summary

Sonneveld, H. M., Strating, M. M., van Staa, A. L., & Nieboer, A. P. (2013). Gaps in transitional care: What are the perceptions of adolescents, parents and providers? *Child: Care, Health and Development, 39*(1), 69–80. https://doi.org/10.1111/j.1365-2214.2011.01354.x

Steele, R. G. (2000). Trajectory of certain death at an unknown time: Children with neurodegenerative life-threatening illnesses. *The Canadian Journal of Nursing Research, 32*(3), 49–67.

Straehla, J. P., Barton, K. S., Yi-Frazier, J. P., Wharton, C., Baker, K. S., Bona, K., Wolfe, J., & Rosenberg, A. R. (2017). The benefits and burdens of cancer: A prospective longitudinal cohort study of adolescents and young adults. *Journal of Palliative Medicine, 20*(5), 494–501. https://doi.org/10.1089/jpm.2016.0369

Suris, J. C., & Parera, N. (2005). Sex, drugs and chronic illness: Health behaviours among chronically ill youth. *European Journal of Public Health, 15*(5), 484–488. https://doi.org/10.1093/eurpub/cki0011

Temel, J. S., Greer, J. A., Muzikansky, A., Gallagher, E. R., Admane, S., Jackson, V. A., Dahlin, C. M., Blinderman, C. D., Jacobsen, J., Pirl, W. F., Billings, J. A., & Lynch, T. J. (2010). Early palliative care for patients with metastatic non-small-cell lung cancer. *The New England Journal of Medicine, 363*(8), 733–742. https://doi.org/10.1056/NEJMoa1000678

Temel, J. S., Greer, J. A., El-Jawahri, A., Pirl, W. F., Park, E. R., Jackson, V. A., Back, A. L., Kamdar, M., Jacobsen, J., Chittenden, E. H., Rinaldi, S. P., Gallagher, E. R., Eusebio, J. R., Li, Z., Muzikansky, A., & Ryan, D. P. (2017). Effects of early integrated palliative care in patients with lung and GI cancer: A randomized clinical trial. *Journal of Clinical Oncology, 35*(8), 834–841. https://doi.org/10.1200/JCO.2016.70.5046

Ullrich, C. K., Rodday, A. M., Bingen, K. M., Kupst, M. J., Patel, S. K., Syrjala, K. L., Harris, L. L., Recklitis, C. J., Chang, G., Guinan, E. C., Terrin, N., Tighiouart, H., Phipps, S., & Parsons, S. K. (2017). Three sides to a story: Child, parent, and nurse perspectives on the child's experience during hematopoietic stem cell transplantation. *Cancer, 123*(16), 3159–3166. https://doi.org/10.1002/cncr.30723

van der Linde, D., Konings, E. E., Slager, M. A., Witsenburg, M., Helbing, W. A., Takkenberg, J. J., & Roos-Hesselink, J. W. (2011). Birth prevalence of congenital heart disease worldwide: A systematic review and meta-analysis. *Journal of the American College of Cardiology, 58*(21), 2241–2247. https://doi.org/10.1016/j.jacc.2011.08.025

Vanopdenbosch, L. J., Maes, E., & Oliver, D. J. (2017). European Academy of Neurology/European Association for Palliative Care Taskforce on Neurology Consensus recommendations on palliative care for patients with chronic and progressive neurological disease—Acceptability for Belgian neurologists. *European Journal of Neurology, 24*(7), 995–998. https://doi.org/10.1111/ene.13325

Vern-Gross, T. Z., Lam, C. G., Graff, Z., Singhal, S., Levine, D. R., Gibson, D., Sykes, A., Anghelescu, D. L., Yuan, Y., & Baker, J. N. (2015). Patterns of end-of-life care in children with advanced solid tumor malignancies enrolled on a palliative care service. *Journal of Pain and Symptom Management, 50*(3), 305–312. https://doi.org/10.1016/j.jpainsymman.2015.03.008

Warren, M. D., McLellan, S. E., Mann, M. Y., Scott, J. A., & Brown, T. W. (2022). Progress, persistence, and hope: Building a system of services for CYSHCN and their families. *Pediatrics, 149*(Suppl 7), e2021056150E. https://doi.org/10.1542/peds.2021-056150E

Weaver, M. S., Heinze, K. E., Kelly, K. P., Wiener, L., Casey, R. L., Bell, C. J., Wolfe, J., Garee, A. M., Watson, A., & Hinds, P. S. (2015). Palliative care as a standard of care in pediatric oncology. *Pediatric Blood & Cancer, 62*(Suppl 5), S829–S833. https://doi.org/10.1002/pbc.25695

Wolfe, J., Grier, H. E., Klar, N., Levin, S. B., Ellenbogen, J. M., Salem-Schatz, S., Emanuel, E. J., & Weeks, J. C. (2000a). Symptoms and suffering at the end of life in children with cancer. *The New England Journal of Medicine, 342*(5), 326–333. https://doi.org/10.1056/NEJM200002033420506

Wolfe, J., Klar, N., Grier, H. E., Duncan, J., Salem-Schatz, S., Emanuel, E. J., & Weeks, J. C. (2000b). Understanding of prognosis among parents of children who died of cancer: Impact on treatment goals and integration of palliative care. *JAMA, 284*(19), 2469–2475. https://doi.org/10.1001/jama.284.19.2469

Wolfe, J., Hammel, J. F., Edwards, K. E., Duncan, J., Comeau, M., Breyer, J., Aldridge, S. A., Grier, H. E., Berde, C., Dussel, V., & Weeks, J. C. (2008). Easing of suffering in children with cancer at the end of life: Is care changing? *Journal of Clinical Oncology, 26*(10), 1717–1723. https://doi.org/10.1200/JCO.2007.14.0277

Wool, C., Côté-Arsenault, D., Perry Black, B., Denney-Koelsch, E., Kim, S., & Kavanaugh, K. (2016). Provision of services in perinatal palliative care: A multicenter survey in the United States. *Journal of Palliative Medicine, 19*(3), 279–285. https://doi.org/10.1089/jpm.2015.0266

World Health Organization (WHO). (2021, November 17). *Mental health of adolescents.* https://www.who.int/news-room/fact-sheets/detail/adolescent-mental-health

World Health Organization (WHO). (n.d.). *Sexual health.* https://www.who.int/health-topics/sexual-health (2024).

Wurm, F., McKeaveney, C., Corr, M., Wilson, A., & Noble, H. (2022). The psychosocial needs of adolescent and young adult kidney transplant recipients, and associated interventions: A scoping review. *BMC Psychology, 10*(1), 186. https://doi.org/10.1186/s40359-022-00893-7

Younge, N., Smith, P. B., Goldberg, R. N., Brandon, D. H., Simmons, C., Cotten, C. M., & Bidegain, M. (2015). Impact of a palliative care program on end-of-life care in a neonatal intensive care unit. *Journal of Perinatology, 35*(3), 218–222. https://doi.org/10.1038/jp.2014.193

Zadeh, S., Pao, M., & Wiener, L. (2015). Opening end-of-life discussions: How to introduce Voicing My CHOiCES™, an advance care planning guide for adolescents and young adults. *Palliative & Supportive Care, 13*(3), 591–599. https://doi.org/10.1017/S1478951514000054

Zalenski, R. J., Jones, S. S., Courage, C., Waselewsky, D. R., Kostaroff, A. S., Kaufman, D., Beemath, A., Brofman, J., Castillo, J. W., Krayem, H., Marinelli, A., Milner, B., Palleschi, M. T., Tareen, M., Testani, S., Soubani, A., Walch, J., Wheeler, J., Wilborn, S., Granovsky, H., et al. (2017). Impact of palliative care screening and consultation in the ICU: A multihospital quality improvement project. *Journal of Pain and Symptom Management, 53*(1), 5–12.e3. https://doi.org/10.1016/j.jpainsymman.2016.08.003

Zhukovsky, D. S., Herzog, C. E., Kaur, G., Palmer, J. L., & Bruera, E. (2009). The impact of palliative care consultation on symptom assessment, communication needs, and palliative interventions in pediatric patients with cancer. *Journal of Palliative Medicine, 12*(4), 343–349. https://doi.org/10.1089/jpm.2008.0152

Zorko, D. J., McNally, J. D., Rochwerg, B., Pinto, N., O'Hearn, K., Almazyad, M. A., Ames, S. G., Brooke, P., Cayouette, F., Chow, C., Coletti, J. J., Francoeur, C., Heneghan, J. A., Kazzaz, Y. M., Killien, E. Y., Jayawarden, S. K., Lasso, R., Lee, L. A., O'Mahony, A., et al. (2023). Defining pediatric chronic critical illness: A scoping review. *Pediatric Critical Care Medicine, 24*(2), e91–e103. https://doi.org/10.1097/PCC.0000000000003125

Chapter 3
Pediatric Palliative Care at End of Life

3.1 Hospice

Hospice care refers to a dedicated branch of palliative care focused on care during the final stages of an individual's life. This type of care is usually offered when prognosis is measured in months, not years. Hospice is a multidisciplinary service that includes medical, spiritual, emotional, and family-focused care with a team of medical providers (physicians, nurse practitioners, nurses, aides), therapists (physical, occupational, music, child life), and psychosocial support (chaplain, social work, volunteer services). Hospice also includes important bereavement support. Hospice care may be delivered in various locations, including a patient's home, nursing facility, hospital, or group home. There are four distinct levels of hospice support that are dependent on clinical need and availability:

1. *Routine Hospice Care*: Routine hospice care delivered in a home setting comprises the majority of hospice care in the United States. The home may be the patient's, a family member's or friend's, or a location that has agreed to house the patient during their hospice care. It is delivered by a multidisciplinary team that meets with the patient in their hospice location and takes over primary care responsibilities for the patient.
2. *Continuous Hospice Care*: Hospice care provided in the home for 8–24 h a day, usually by nurses with the help of aides and guidance of medical providers. As its name indicates, this is a designation for patients requiring continuous interventions. This is useful, short-term support for severe symptom management and moments requiring close observation.
3. *Inpatient Respite Care*: This type of hospice care is arranged to provide respite for home providers. Many families are caring for their loved ones without additional help, and the burden of care can be overwhelming. Hospices can contract

C. Delgado-Corcoran et al., *Specialized Pediatric Palliative Care*,
SpringerBriefs in Public Health, https://doi.org/10.1007/978-3-031-65452-7_3

with local facilities for ongoing medical care in a supervised setting for 5 days or less. This can allow a patient's loved ones to take care of other needs and have some restoration before coming back to full-time caregiving.

4. *General Inpatient Care*: Inpatient hospitalization for ongoing hospice support is usually due to needs so severe that they must be attended to with the resources of an inpatient setting. Often, though not always, the reason for a transition to general inpatient care is uncontrolled physical symptoms that require intensive interventions and close observation. This can occur in a hospital, dedicated hospice, or nursing facility. This type of care has become more common over the past 10 years, though it continues to be a small minority of hospice work done in the United States, and in pediatric hospitals it remains an extremely rare occurrence.

Pediatric hospice teams are dedicated pediatric professionals with training and expertise in caring for children and their families at the end of life. They are often embedded or work closely with hospital-based pediatric palliative care teams. Pediatric hospice and palliative medicine is a young specialty that bears its origins in the adult hospice movement, and to this day most children receive hospice services from community-based adult programs (National Hospice and Palliative Care Organization [NHPCO], 2023). The need for a dedicated pediatric palliative field rose from clinicians and researchers realizing that children were dying with significant symptom burden, often not addressing their "total" pain and distress. Early pediatric palliative care (PPC) clinical and academic work, starting in the 1970s and rapidly expanding by the 2000s, focused on supporting the dying child (Sisk et al., 2020). Pediatric palliative care has since grown to include lifelong support of children with serious illnesses, but hospice care remains a core pillar of PPC. Access to pediatric hospice continues to have significant limitations and barriers even though many patients and providers express preferences for the home for end-of-life care (Kassam et al., 2014). Most patients are referred by pediatric subspecialists or palliative care teams. Children who do receive pediatric hospice care most often have genetic or oncological diagnoses (NHPCO, 2023). Neuromuscular and neurodegenerative conditions make up the next two most common conditions. Interestingly, pediatric hospice patients tend to have a shorter length of stay in hospice compared to adults (NHPCO, 2023).

There is significant variety in the geographic availability of hospice services. More than half of children's hospitals report not having access to dedicated pediatric hospice services (Weaver et al., 2022). In fact, that number has continued to decline (NHPCO, 2023). As such, of the children receiving dedicated hospice services, most are under the care of adult hospice providers (Lindley & Shaw, 2014; Lindley & Edwards, 2015). It is estimated that over half of hospice agencies do not have a dedicated pediatric team, and 71.5% of counties in the United States do not have an available home-based pediatric hospice team (NHPCO, 2023). Many hospices are required to contract out to provide pediatric dedicated care (NHPCO, 2023). This lends itself to tremendous variability in access, experience, and quality.

3.2 Concurrent Care

While concurrent hospice and therapeutic care has expanded support, there are still many children and families who must decide between hospice support and disease-directed therapy. In an effort to improve access to end-of-life hospice care for children, the 2010 Patient Protection and Affordable Care Act (ACA) provisioned the Concurrent Care Act (section 2302), which mandates that Medicaid and Children's Health Insurance Programs (CHIP) cover the hospice benefit for children under the age of 21 with a hospice-certifiable diagnosis while they continue to undergo curative treatment. This guarantees that children under the age of 21 who have a terminal diagnosis but are still pursuing disease-directed therapy, such as chemotherapy or radiation, can continue to receive both services. Concurrent care is covered by Medicaid, CHIP, and TRICARE; however, there is no provision within the ACA that requires private insurance to cover concurrent care. Few national insurance companies will cover this benefit automatically, and private insurance accounts for only 32% of pediatric hospice reimbursement coverages (NHPCO, 2023). Some private insurances will offer concurrent care coverage on a case-by-case basis through a "carve-out." This often requires significant administrative arrangements and is not guaranteed.

3.3 Impact of Pediatric Palliative Care at End of Life

In instances where a pediatric patient is approaching end of life, providing high-quality, comfort-focused care for both the patient and their family is of the utmost importance (Linebarger et al., 2022; Norris et al., 2019). Patients may experience physical suffering, and both the patient and their family may face significant emotional and spiritual distress. Patients in their final days require careful symptom management, and families may need extra support as death approaches (Harman & Walling, 2023). For families, PPC involvement at end of life improves goal-concordant care and parental satisfaction with care, decreases anxiety and decisional regret, and improves coping and bereavement outcomes. For patients, PPC involvement improves satisfaction with care, symptom management, and quality of life while decreasing the frequency of painful and invasive procedures. PPC involvement has also been shown to result in cost savings surrounding end-of-life care (Lo et al., 2022; Chong et al., 2018). In a study comparing the experiences of children at the end of life with and without palliative care support, those receiving palliative services had fewer invasive interventions, median inpatient days, and deaths in the intensive care setting (Keele et al., 2013).

3.3.1 Decision-Making, Goal Concordance, and Emotional Support

In end-of-life situations, shared decision-making, which is a hallmark of pediatric palliative care, is especially valuable (Linebarger et al., 2022; Norris et al., 2019). Current guidance for pediatric end-of-life care includes anticipatory counseling regarding the dying process (Linebarger et al., 2022). The interdisciplinary approach to palliative care provided by team members with experience in end-of-life care allows for the provision of this counseling in a developmentally appropriate manner that is tailored to the unique needs and preferences of pediatric patients and their families (Linebarger et al., 2022; Johnston et al., 2017).

Referrals to pediatric palliative care provide families with an initial opportunity to share preferences regarding the location of death and goals of end-of-life care (Mitchell et al., 2017). Patients who engage with PPC have more frequent advance care planning discussions and resuscitation status documentation (Moynihan et al., 2021; Kaye et al., 2021). In one study, almost 80% of young adult cancer patients receiving palliative care had a do-not-resuscitate order in place, even when palliative care was consulted within days of death (Mark et al., 2019; Keim-Malpass et al., 2014). Similarly, families of young people hospitalized in a CICU study had advance care planning at twice the frequency as families not receiving palliative care (Moynihan et al., 2021).

Families receiving specialized pediatric palliative care services noted greater satisfaction with overall care. They indicated that care planning and emotional support contributed to this satisfaction (Mitchell et al., 2017). These families received support with decision-making processes, particularly communicating with their children and other care team members. The involvement of PPC in the pediatric intensive care unit (PICU) decreases the likelihood of parental anxiety, depression, and regret and facilitates shared decision-making (Cuviello et al., 2022; Mitchell et al., 2017). In a survey of families whose children received end-of-life palliative care at one hospital, most respondents agreed that PPC helped set goals and that those goals were met and supported (Sheetz & Bowman, 2013).

3.3.2 Symptom Management and Quality of Life

A primary goal of palliative care is to alleviate, if not fully eliminate, the burden of distressing symptoms. As such, this is a common reason for referral to specialist pediatric palliative teams (Mitchell et al., 2017; Kaye et al., 2021). Evidence suggests that the involvement of pediatric palliative care improves symptom management and quality of life at end of life. Parents have reported that symptom management improved following the introduction of palliative services and that symptoms were well controlled at end of life (Mitchell et al., 2017; Sheetz & Bowman, 2013). In a sample of 114 children who died in an inpatient hospital setting, those who received an inpatient PPC consult experienced both greater rates of pain assessments and more frequent documentation of pain management plans than those without a consult (Osenga et al., 2016). It has also been shown that young people with cancer have lower pain scores after referral to PPC and increased use of medications to manage pain (Kaye et al., 2018). Additionally, children hospitalized in a CICU and receiving palliative support were more often awake and being administered enteral feeds than those not receiving palliative care (Moynihan et al., 2021). Finally, home-based PPC involvement among pediatric oncology patients was found to significantly increase quality-of-life indicators, including having fun and experiencing an event that added meaning to their lives (Friedrichsdorf et al., 2015).

3.3.3 Frequency of Invasive Procedures and Interventions

Involvement of PPC also appears to impact the frequency of painful or invasive procedures initiated at end of life. Among pediatric patients who died in an inpatient hospital setting, those with a PPC consult were significantly less likely to experience potentially painful monitoring procedures including blood draws and intravenous line placements in the last 48 h of life. Additionally, those children with a PPC consult were more likely to have a do-not-resuscitate order in place at the time of their death, allowing them to avoid potentially unsuccessful resuscitative attempts that are not desired by the patient and/or their family (Osenga et al., 2016). Participants in home-based care have been shown to have decreased rates of high-intensity therapies such as total parenteral nutrition, cardioversion, hemodialysis, invasive monitoring, mechanical ventilation, and surgeries (Lo et al., 2022).

Although there is limited data examining the role of PPC in end-of-life care in children with heart disease (Delgado-Corcoran et al., 2020; Moynihan et al., 2021; Morell et al., 2019), there are some studies that demonstrate the added value of PPC involvement in the care of children in the cardiac intensive care unit (CICU). In a sample of 218 deceased children who received care in the CICU and died, children without a documented PPC consult were significantly more likely to experience the initiation of invasive procedures in the last 14 days of life (Songer et al., 2023). In a single-center study, Moynihan et al. (2021) found that patients in the CICU who were receiving palliative services had lower rates of mechanical ventilation, extracorporeal membrane oxygenation, cardiopulmonary resuscitation, and inotrope administration (Moynihan et al., 2021). In the same study, those without palliative care support were three times more likely to receive cardiopulmonary resuscitation in the week prior to death (Moynihan et al., 2021).

Delgado-Corcoran et al. (2020) noted that PPC involvement in the CICU occurred infrequently in the setting of high disease burden, complexity, and lower survival. However, PPC was associated with more frequent use of comfort care at the end of life and death at home (Delgado-Corcoran et al., 2020). These studies showed PPC involvement in approximately half of the deaths and a median time to consultation prior to death of 60 days. The low rate of PPC involvement in children with cardiac issues differs from the data in children with cancer, where more than 75% of children who died had PPC involvement more than 30 days prior to death, and the overall median time between consultation and death was >100 days. Oncology data suggests dramatic reductions in the intensity of medical therapy at end of life with PPC involvement while also indicating some disparities in PPC utilization according to social determinants of health (DeWitt et al., 2020; Snaman et al., 2017; Kaye et al., 2018). Cancer patients without palliative care were more than twice as likely to undergo invasive measures (Jewitt et al., 2023). A US study in young cancer patients showed fewer ICU deaths and less intensive treatments overall for patients with specialized palliative care support (Snaman et al., 2017). Children and young adults receiving cancer treatment in France have also demonstrated decreased incidence of high-intensity treatment when receiving palliative care services (Jewitt et al., 2023), and one Canadian study observed a 50% increase in the receipt of high-intensity care at end of life among cancer patients without palliative care support (Jewitt et al., 2023).

However, it is important to recognize that the ultimate goal is not to limit care at the end of life but to demonstrate concordance with informed advance care planning, and escalated treatments may be part of a palliative care plan. An example of this is noninvasive mechanical ventilation, which, in a study described by Keele et al. (2013), was administered to participants with and without palliative support at similar rates.

3.3.4   Care Setting at End of Life

A recent review of literature showed that most families would prefer to have their child's end of life at home (Walker et al., 2023). Privacy, physical closeness, a comforting environment, and the ability to attend to important practices or rituals were identified as valued benefits (Walker et al., 2023). Family stress associated with receiving care in a pediatric intensive care unit has been documented (O'Meara et al., 2022; Alzawad et al., 2021). Sights and sounds, procedures, behaviors of professionals, appearance and behavior of their child, communication with staff, and difficulty with parental role have been identified as stressors by parents of children in the ICU (Alzawad et al., 2021). Further, parents of deceased children have shared that processes involved in intensive care made involvement in their child's care and memory-making difficult (Broden et al., 2022). These difficulties are an unintended result of the intensive care environment, which can necessitate sedation, safe positioning, timed treatments, and proximity to equipment at the expense of family closeness. Though the optimal setting for care is the one that is most aligned with a family's goals, death outside of an intensive care setting is sometimes considered a quality measure.

Location of death is impacted by PPC involvement, with this finding occurring in various specialties, including oncology and cardiology. Among children treated in a CICU prior to their death, those children without a documented PPC consult died in the ICU more frequently than those with a documented PPC consult (Songer et al., 2023). In some studies, children with cancer receiving palliative care were more likely to have a documented preferred location of death, and to have more time at home near end of life (Kaye et al., 2021). One such study reported that children with cancer who received concurrent end-of-life care via a PPC home care program were significantly more likely to die at home than those children who did not (Friedrichsdorf et al., 2015). Another study involving a sample of 321 pediatric oncology patients noted that a specialized palliative care consultation more than 30 days prior to end of life correlated with a fivefold decrease in the likelihood of intensive care admission (Kaye et al., 2021). While 21% of dying young people receiving palliative care in the study died in the PICU, 72% of those without palliative care died in the intensive care unit (Keele et al., 2013). This suggests that the timing of PPC involvement may be uniquely impactful in helping patients experience end of life outside of the ICU (Kaye et al., 2018). These findings are consistent with current pediatric end-of-life care guidelines that encourage early involvement of PPC as early initiation allows for rapport building, anticipatory support, and planning (Lo et al., 2022; Linebarger et al., 2022).

A factor in families' decision-making regarding care setting is their sense of competency; caregivers who are confident that they will be able to provide sufficient care are more likely to elect for care at home (Walker et al., 2023). One study noted that caregivers of young people with chronic illnesses were more likely to feel confident in their ability to provide care for their child in the home setting, while parents of young people with cancer felt less prepared to do so (Broden et al., 2022). Palliative care support can include assessing family members' comfort with necessary medical care, communicating education needs, providing education resources, and recognizing and honoring established skills. These interventions are particularly helpful for families that have identified home as the desired setting for their child's end-of-life care.

Of note, very few studies include perspectives of young people themselves regarding care setting. In a study by Taylor et al. (2021), children were more concerned that care assured them familiar providers and adequate time with them, as well as respectful treatment, than they were in the setting of care.

3.3.5   Cost of Care

Cost savings surrounding end-of-life care are observed when palliative services are involved (Lo et al., 2022; Chong et al., 2018). Some studies have shown lower median and average daily charges over the course of hospitalization (Keele et al., 2013). Children and young adults hospitalized in a cardiac intensive care unit receiving palliative care had decreased health care costs for the 7 days prior to death (Moynihan et al., 2021). A study of home-based care in Singapore showed cost savings of 70% in the last year of life and 87% in the last month of life for young people receiving palliative care (Chong et al., 2018). In a comparison of young Canadian patients who qualified for a palliative care referral, estimated costs savings for those receiving palliative care was $9,053,220 per year (Lysecki et al., 2022). Finally, a US-based home PPC program maintaining a census of 20–30 patients showed decreased emergency department utilization and estimated median annual cost avoidance of $110,300 (Mastro et al., 2015).

3.3.6 Conclusions

Research certainly demonstrates a significant positive impact of PPC on end-of-life care. However, there is much work still to be done. Current end-of-life quality measures are adult-focused and fail to address the unique aspects of pediatric end-of-life care, highlighting the need for the creation and validation of pediatric-specific end-of-life quality measures (Johnston et al., 2017). While data suggests adults prefer to die at home, the data among pediatric patients is more variable (Linebarger et al., 2022; Johnston et al., 2017). In-hospital pediatric death is a complicated and challenging phenomenon. As opposed to adult medicine, for which in-hospital death, ICU admission near death, and little to no hospice involvement are considered indicators of poor-quality end-of-life care, this is not the case in pediatric medicine (Johnston et al., 2017). Many factors determine in-hospital versus home death in the pediatric population; these include the patient's condition, sense of security in the hospital setting, concerns of symptom control outside the hospital, impact of home death on siblings, delayed PPC referral, and the lack of centers offering pediatric-focused palliative and hospice care (Johnston et al., 2017; Dussel et al., 2009; Kassam et al., 2014).

In short, while evidence suggests PPC involvement is promotive of high-quality end-of-life care, additional research and development are required to ensure quality indicators are applicable to the unique stressors and experiences associated with pediatric end-of-life care.

3.4 Bereavement Support for Health Care Providers

Caring for a dying child or adolescent is uniquely distressing due in part to the relative rarity of these occurrences and the potential for the death of a child to be viewed as unnatural (Contro et al., 2004). Aspects of care that have been identified as distressing by health care staff who have experienced the death of a young patient include the long-term relationship shared with the patient and family, the provision of aggressive medical treatment during a patient's death, unexpected deaths, conflict with family, and differing cultural values or practices (Keene et al., 2010). When a child or adolescent dies, the impact of this loss is felt by their entire care team across the continuum of care (Linebarger et al., 2022). These experiences of grief are unique to the individual experiencing them (Linebarger et al., 2022) and include psychological and spiritual needs (Copeland & Liska, 2016). When these experiences of grief go unprocessed and these needs are unmet, the well-being of the staff member is at risk (Dryden-Palmer et al., 2018), highlighting the importance of targeted interventions to assist staff members in expressing and coping with their grief.

National guidelines for pediatric end-of-life care include the provision of opportunities for the interdisciplinary PPC team to debrief experiences involving the death of a patient (Linebarger et al., 2022). Current guidelines for PPC include the proactive evaluation of the psychological and spiritual needs of health care professionals and addressing those needs via group debriefings, psychological and spiritual counseling, peer-to-peer support, and educational programs (AAP, 2013).

Current programming that allows staff to debrief, honor the deceased, and process their grief varies across institutions and includes the utilization of a post-code pause (Copeland & Liska, 2016) and rounding on the patient the day following their death (Morrison & Madrigal, 2020). Structured debriefing sessions provided for the deceased child's multidisciplinary care team and facilitated by a trained individual have been utilized in several institutions and are endorsed by participants as being helpful (Delgado-Corcoran et al., 2024; Bateman et al., 2012; Wintermeyer-Pingel et al., 2013). Specific aspects of these sessions identified by participants as valuable include their timeliness, consistency, and inclusion of the multidisciplinary team (Delgado-Corcoran et al., 2024; Bateman et al., 2012).

Current clinical practice guidelines for oncology palliative care include interventions to support health care professionals after the death of a patient such as the fostering of a safe environment for staff to discuss patient deaths and the provision of support in the emotional response to their patient's death (Wintermeyer-Pingel et al., 2013). In one institution, interdisciplinary bereavement debriefing sessions facilitated by a member of the PPC team were described by over 95% of 184 attendees and survey respondents as helpful, informative, and meaningful (Rushton et al., 2006).

Experiencing the death of a pediatric patient is understandably distressing and may evoke a variety of feelings among the care team. Bereavement debriefing sessions and programs provide health care professionals with an opportunity to honor their deceased patients and express and learn to cope with their grief.

References

Alzawad, Z., Marcus Lewis, F., Ngo, L., & Thomas, K. (2021). Exploratory model of parental stress during children's hospitalisation in a paediatric intensive care unit. *Intensive & Critical Care Nursing, 67*, 103109. https://doi.org/10.1016/j.iccn.2021.103109

American Academy of Pediatrics (AAP), Section on Hospice and Palliative Medicine and Committee on Hospital Care. (2013). Pediatric palliative care and hospice care commitments, guidelines, and recommendations. *Pediatrics, 132*(5), 966–972. https://doi.org/10.1542/peds.2013-2731

Bateman, S. T., Dixon, R., & Trozzi, M. (2012). The wrap-up: A unique forum to support pediatric residents when faced with the death of a child. *Journal of Palliative Medicine, 15*(12), 1329–1334. https://doi.org/10.1089/jpm.2012.0253

Broden, E. G., Hinds, P. S., Werner-Lin, A. V., & Curley, M. A. Q. (2022). "I didn't want my baby to pass, but I didn't want him suffering either": Comparing bereaved parents' narratives with nursing end-of-life assessments in the pediatric intensive care unit. *Journal of Hospice & Palliative Nursing, 24*(5), 271–280. https://doi.org/10.1097/NJH.0000000000000884

Chong, P. H., De Castro Molina, J. A., Teo, K., & Tan, W. S. (2018). Paediatric palliative care improves patient outcomes and reduces healthcare costs: Evaluation of a home-based program. *BMC Palliative Care, 17*(1), 11. https://doi.org/10.1186/s12904-017-0267-z

Contro, N. A., Larson, J., Scofield, S., Sourkes, B., & Cohen, H. J. (2004). Hospital staff and family perspectives regarding quality of pediatric palliative care. *Pediatrics, 114*(5), 1248–1252. https://doi.org/10.1542/peds.2003-0857-L

Copeland, D., & Liska, H. (2016). Implementation of a post-code pause: Extending post-event debriefing to include silence. *Journal of Trauma Nursing, 23*(2), 58–64. https://doi.org/10.1097/JTN.0000000000000187

Cuviello, A., Pasli, M., Hurley, C., Bhatia, S., Anghelescu, D. L., & Baker, J. N. (2022). Compassionate de-escalation of life-sustaining treatments in pediatric oncology: An opportunity for palliative care and intensive care collaboration. *Frontiers in Oncology, 12*, 1017272. https://doi.org/10.3389/fonc.2022.1017272

Delgado-Corcoran, C., Wawrzynski, S. E., Bennett, E. E., Green, D., Bodily, S., Moore, D., Cook, L. J., & Olson, L. M. (2020). Palliative care in children with heart disease treated in an ICU. *Pediatric Critical Care Medicine, 21*(5), 423–429. https://doi.org/10.1097/PCC.0000000000002271

Delgado-Corcoran, C., Wawrzynski, S. E., Mansfield, K., Fuchs, E., Yeates, C., Flaherty, B. F., Harousseau, M., Cook, L., & Epps, J. V. (2024). Grieving children' death in an intensive care unit: Implementation of a standardized process. *Journal of Palliative Medicine, 27*(2), 236–240. https://doi.org/10.1089/jpm.2023.0134

DeWitt, A. G., Rossano, J. W., Bailly, D. K., Bhat, P. N., Chanani, N. K., Kirkland, B. W., Moga, M. A., Owens, G. E., Retzloff, L. B., Zhang, W., Banerjee, M., Costarino, A. T., Bird, G. L., & Gaies, M. (2020). Predicting and surviving prolonged critical illness after congenital heart surgery. *Critical Care Medicine, 48*(7), e557–e564. https://doi.org/10.1097/CCM.0000000000004354

Dryden-Palmer, K., Garros, D., Meyer, E. C., Farrell, C., & Parshuram, C. S. (2018). Care for dying children and their families in the PICU: Promoting clinician education, support, and resilience. *Pediatric Critical Care Medicine, 19*(8S Suppl 2), S79–S85. https://doi.org/10.1097/PCC.0000000000001594

Dussel, V., Kreicbergs, U., Hilden, J. M., Watterson, J., Moore, C., Turner, B. G., Weeks, J. C., & Wolfe, J. (2009). Looking beyond where children die: Determinants and effects of planning a child's location of death. *Journal of Pain and Symptom Management, 37*(1), 33–43. https://doi.org/10.1016/j.jpainsymman.2007.12.017

Friedrichsdorf, S. J., Postier, A., Dreyfus, J., Osenga, K., Sencer, S., & Wolfe, J. (2015). Improved quality of life at end of life related to home-based palliative care in children with cancer. *Journal of Palliative Medicine, 18*(2), 143–150. https://doi.org/10.1089/jpm.2014.0285

Harman, S. M., & Walling, A. M. (2023, August 24). *Palliative care: The last hours and days of life.* UpToDate. Retrieved March 13, 2024, from https://www.uptodate.com/contents/palliative-care-the-last-hours-and-days-of-life

Jewitt, N., Rapoport, A., Gupta, A., Srikanthan, A., Sutradhar, R., Luo, J., Widger, K., Wolfe, J., Earle, C. C., Gupta, S., & Kassam, A. (2023). The effect of specialized palliative care on end-of-life care intensity in AYAs with cancer. *Journal of Pain and Symptom Management, 65*(3), 222–232. https://doi.org/10.1016/j.jpainsymman.2022.11.013

Johnston, E. E., Rosenberg, A. R., & Kamal, A. H. (2017). Pediatric-specific end-of-life care quality measures: An unmet need of a vulnerable population. *Journal of Oncology Practice, 13*(10), e874–e880. https://doi.org/10.1200/JOP.2017.021766

Kassam, A., Skiadaresis, J., Alexander, S., & Wolfe, J. (2014). Parent and clinician preferences for location of end-of-life care: Home, hospital or freestanding hospice? *Pediatric Blood & Cancer, 61*(5), 859–864. https://doi.org/10.1002/pbc.24872

Kaye, E. C., Gushue, C. A., DeMarsh, S., Jerkins, J., Sykes, A., Lu, Z., Snaman, J. M., Blazin, L., Johnson, L. M., Levine, D. R., Morrison, R. R., & Baker, J. N. (2018). Illness and end-of-life experiences of children with cancer who receive palliative care. *Pediatric Blood & Cancer, 65*(4). https://doi.org/10.1002/pbc.26895

Kaye, E. C., Weaver, M. S., DeWitt, L. H., Byers, E., Stevens, S. E., Lukowski, J., Shih, B., Zalud, K., Applegarth, J., Wong, H. N., Baker, J. N., Ullrich, C. K., & AAHPM Research Committee. (2021). The impact of specialty palliative care in pediatric oncology: A systematic review. *Journal of Pain and Symptom Management, 61*(5), 1060–1079.e2. https://doi.org/10.1016/j.jpainsymman.2020.12.003

Keele, L., Keenan, H. T., Sheetz, J., & Bratton, S. L. (2013). Differences in characteristics of dying children who receive and do not receive palliative care. *Pediatrics, 132*(1), 72–78. https://doi.org/10.1542/peds.2013-0470

Keene, E. A., Hutton, N., Hall, B., & Rushton, C. (2010). Bereavement debriefing sessions: An intervention to support health care professionals in managing their grief after the death of a patient. *Pediatric Nursing, 36*(4), 185–189.

Keim-Malpass, J., Erickson, J. M., & Malpass, H. C. (2014). End-of-life care characteristics for young adults with cancer who die in the hospital. *Journal of Palliative Medicine, 17*(12), 1359–1364. https://doi.org/10.1089/jpm.2013.0661

Lindley, L. C., & Edwards, S. L. (2015). Geographic access to hospice care for children with cancer in Tennessee, 2009 to 2011. *American Journal of Hospice & Palliative Care, 32*(8), 849–854. https://doi.org/10.1177/1049909114543641

Lindley, L. C., & Shaw, S. L. (2014). Who are the children using hospice care? *Journal for Specialists in Pediatric Nursing, 19*(4), 308–315. https://doi.org/10.1111/jspn.12085

Linebarger, J. S., Johnson, V., Boss, R. D., & Section on Hospice and Palliative Medicine. (2022). Guidance for pediatric end-of-life care. *Pediatrics, 149*(5), e2022057011. https://doi.org/10.1542/peds.2022-057011

Lo, D. S., Hein, N., & Bulgareli, J. V. (2022). Pediatric palliative care and end-of-life: A systematic review of economic health analyses. *Revista Paulista de Pediatria, 40*, e2021002. https://doi.org/10.1590/1984-0462/2022/40/2021002

Lysecki, D. L., Gupta, S., Rapoport, A., Rhodes, E., Spruin, S., Vadeboncoeur, C., Widger, K., & Tanuseputro, P. (2022). Children's health care utilization and cost in the last year of life: A cohort comparison with and without regional specialist pediatric palliative care. *Journal of Palliative Medicine, 25*(7), 1031–1040. https://doi.org/10.1089/jpm.2021.0175

Mark, M. S. J., Yang, G., Ding, L., Norris, R. E., & Thienprayoon, R. (2019). Location of death and end-of-life characteristics of young adults with cancer treated at a pediatric hospital. *Journal of Adolescent and Young Adult Oncology, 8*(4), 417–422. https://doi.org/10.1089/jayao.2018.0123

Mastro, K. A., Johnson, J. E., McElvery, N., & Preuster, C. (2015). The benefits of a nurse-driven, patient- and family-centered pediatric palliative care program. *The Journal of Nursing Administration, 45*(9), 423–428. https://doi.org/10.1097/NNA.0000000000000227

Mitchell, S., Morris, A., Bennett, K., Sajid, L., & Dale, J. (2017). Specialist paediatric palliative care services: What are the benefits? *Archives of Disease in Childhood, 102*(10), 923–929. https://doi.org/10.1136/archdischild-2016-312026

Morell, E., Moynihan, K., Wolfe, J., & Blume, E. D. (2019). Palliative care and paediatric cardiology: Current evidence and future directions. *The Lancet Child & Adolescent Health, 3*(7), 502–510. https://doi.org/10.1016/S2352-4642(19)30121-X

Morrison, W., & Madrigal, V. (2020). We still round the next day. *Pediatrics, 145*(3), e20192035. https://doi.org/10.1542/peds.2019-2035

Moynihan, K. M., Heith, C. S., Snaman, J. M., Smith-Parrish, M., Bakas, A., Ge, S., Cerqueira, A. V., Bailey, V., Beke, D., Wolfe, J., Morell, E., Gauvreau, K., & Blume, E. D. (2021). Palliative care referrals in cardiac disease. *Pediatrics, 147*(3), e2020018580. https://doi.org/10.1542/peds.2020-018580

National Hospice and Palliative Care Organization (NHPCO). (2023). *NHPCO pediatric facts and figures* (23rd ed.). National Hospice and Palliative Care Organization. https://www.nhpco.org/wp-content/uploads/NHPCO_Pediatric_Facts_Figures_2023.pdf

Norris, S., Minkowitz, S., & Scharbach, K. (2019). Pediatric palliative care. *Primary Care, 46*(3), 461–473. https://doi.org/10.1016/j.pop.2019.05.010

O'Meara, A., Akande, M., Yagiela, L., Hummel, K., Whyte-Nesfield, M., Michelson, K. N., Radman, M., Traube, C., Manning, J. C., & Hartman, M. E. (2022). Family outcomes after the pediatric intensive care unit: A scoping review. *Journal of Intensive Care Medicine, 37*(9), 1179–1198. https://doi.org/10.1177/08850666211056603

Osenga, K., Postier, A., Dreyfus, J., Foster, L., Teeple, W., & Friedrichsdorf, S. J. (2016). A comparison of circumstances at the end of life in a hospital setting for children with palliative care involvement versus those without. *Journal of Pain and Symptom Management, 52*(5), 673–680. https://doi.org/10.1016/j.jpainsymman.2016.05.024

Rushton, C. H., Reder, E., Hall, B., Comello, K., Sellers, D. E., & Hutton, N. (2006). Interdisciplinary interventions to improve pediatric palliative care and reduce health care professional suffering. *Journal of Palliative Medicine, 9*(4), 922–933. https://doi.org/10.1089/jpm.2006.9.922

Sheetz, M. J., & Bowman, M. A. (2013). Parents' perceptions of a pediatric palliative program. *American Journal of Hospice & Palliative Care, 30*(3), 291–296. https://doi.org/10.1177/1049909112449376

Sisk, B. A., Feudtner, C., Bluebond-Langner, M., Sourkes, B., Hinds, P. S., & Wolfe, J. (2020). Response to suffering of the seriously ill child: A history of palliative care for children. *Pediatrics, 145*(1), e20191741. https://doi.org/10.1542/peds.2019-1741

Snaman, J. M., Kaye, E. C., Lu, J. J., Sykes, A., & Baker, J. N. (2017). Palliative care involvement is associated with less intensive end-of-life care in adolescent and young adult oncology patients. *Journal of Palliative Medicine, 20*(5), 509–516. https://doi.org/10.1089/jpm.2016.0451

Songer, K., Wawrzynski, S. E., Olson, L., & Delgado-Corcoran, C. (2023, August 27–September 1). *Effect of timing of palliative care consultation on end-of-life care for children with advanced cardiac disease.* [Poster presentation]. 8th World congress of pediatric cardiology and cardiac surgery, Washington, DC, USA. https://www.wcpccs2023.org/event/1da8563e-0f65-486c-88df-70c3db431af5/summary

Taylor, J., Murphy, S., Chambers, L., & Aldridge, J. (2021). Consulting with young people: Informing guidelines for children's palliative care. *Archives of Disease in Childhood, 106*(7), 693–697. https://doi.org/10.1136/archdischild-2020-320353

Walker, M., Nicolardi, D., Christopoulos, T., & Ross, T. (2023). Hospital, hospice, or home: A scoping review of the importance of place in pediatric palliative care. *Palliative & Supportive Care, 21*(5), 925–934. https://doi.org/10.1017/S1478951523000664

Weaver, M. S., Shostrom, V. K., Kaye, E. C., Keegan, A., & Lindley, L. C. (2022). Palliative care programs in children's hospitals. *Pediatrics, 150*(4), e2022057872. https://doi.org/10.1542/peds.2022-057872

Wintermeyer-Pingel, S. A., Murphy, D., & Hammelef, K. J. (2013). Improving a grief and loss program: Caring for patients, families, and staff. *Omega (Westport), 67*(1–2), 233–239. https://doi.org/10.2190/OM.67.1-2.z3

Chapter 4
Accessing Pediatric Palliative Care

4.1 Nationwide Availability of Specialized Pediatric Palliative Care

While access to pediatric palliative care (PPC) has expanded since its initial recognition by the American Board of Medical Specialties in 2006, research indicates substantial variability regarding the staffing, funding, and services provided by PPC programs across the United States (Feudtner et al., 2013). Factors contributing to the variability of composition across sites include the amount of time a PPC program has been in place and funding sources for the program. A 2022 survey of 148 hospitals identified that 20% of respondents still did not have a PPC program, and over half of the facilities reported not having access to pediatric hospice or respite care (Weaver et al., 2022). Furthermore, these PPC programs are located predominantly in urban areas at larger academic centers, with much less access in rural areas (Rogers & Kirch, 2019). Many barriers exist to equitable access to PPC both within the United States and globally, including family and provider perceptions of palliative care, funding and insurance limitations, staffing and education deficits, as well as barriers rooted in bias related to culture, language, and race/ethnicity.

4.1.1 Composition of Specialized Pediatric Palliative Care Teams Across the United States

The establishment of PPC programs began in the late 1990s and early 2000s (Feudtner et al., 2013). Today, PPC programs must continue to evolve to meet the dynamic needs of patients and families. An interdisciplinary team approach to PPC allows for care that meets the unique physical, psychosocial, and spiritual needs of

© The Author(s), under exclusive license to Springer Nature Switzerland AG 2024
C. Delgado-Corcoran et al., *Specialized Pediatric Palliative Care*,
SpringerBriefs in Public Health, https://doi.org/10.1007/978-3-031-65452-7_4

patients and their families (Norris et al., 2019; Bergstraesser, 2013). The American Academy of Pediatrics (AAP, 2013) recommends that PPC teams include physicians, nurses, social workers, case managers, spiritual care providers, bereavement specialists, and child life specialists. Newer PPC programs may start with only a few team members and grow over time (AAP, 2013).

While variability exists in the composition of PPC teams across the United States, research on the topic indicates many programs report their team including the following roles: physician, advanced practice registered nurse and/or nurse practitioner, social worker, registered nurse, and chaplain (Feudtner et al., 2013; Weaver et al., 2018; Rogers et al., 2021; Keele et al., 2016). Additional roles reported to varying levels may include a child life specialist, bereavement coordinator, administrative assistant, therapist (representing art, music, physical and occupational therapy, among others), pharmacist, and psychologist (Feudtner et al., 2013; Weaver et al., 2018; Rogers et al., 2021). In a sample of 44 PPC directors and hospital administrators, researchers found that both the number of team members on the PPC team and the number of hospitals with a larger PPC team increased over time (Keele et al., 2016). This suggests that the composition of PPC teams may grow and change with time and the maturation of programs. Research findings regarding the impact of PPC team composition on the number of PPC consultations are mixed (Feudtner et al., 2013; Keele et al., 2016). Additional research on longitudinal changes to the composition of PPC teams and the impact of team composition on the frequency of PPC consultations is warranted.

4.2   Inpatient Pediatric Palliative Care

The roots of PPC lie primarily in large academic children's hospitals with a concentrated—though not exclusive—focus on inpatient care. Early pioneers and most currently existing programs first found their home in hospitals, often affiliating themselves with a related academic division that focuses on inpatient care such as critical care, oncology, hospitalist medicine, or anesthesia. The alignment was often determined by local dynamics, budgets, and individual champions of palliative care as a specialty of value (Sisk et al., 2020).

As the medical subspecialty has evolved, it has quickly become a central part of the quality of care in US hospitals. Availability of palliative care is now considered a benchmark of a high-quality children's hospital and individual program excellence in rankings such as US News and World Report. Specialties such as critical care, hospital medicine, oncology, and cardiology find that the presence of a robust palliative care program can be a major asset as they work to recruit providers from a competitive pool of applicants. The attention to and advocacy for quality palliative care have played a role in highlighting the value of these programs, which tend to be revenue negative and rely on supplemental help through the hospital's operating budget or philanthropic funds to operate. Inpatient palliative care has a range of proven benefits for both children and adults, though in children we find that some of these benefits hold different weight compared with adult programs. Adult inpatient hospitals find a proven benefit not only in higher quality of care for grown patients, but also in length of stay, mortality measurements, and readmission rates—factors that carry different regulatory and resource benefits in children (Srinivasan et al., 2023). In our current operating models for children's hospitals, some of these benefits are either not measurable or not impactful to a degree that they are a primary motivator for decisions about funding these operations. This dynamic partially explains the data suggesting that pediatric palliative care has continued to significantly favor large metropolitan areas and large academic medical centers. In the National Hospice and Palliative Care Organization's (NHPCO) data for pediatric palliative care nationwide, inpatient-based palliative care was provided in 15.8% of nonmetropolitan counties and 23% of metropolitan counties.

Less than half (48%) of the organizations who responded to the NHPCO's Needs Assessment have a dedicated pediatric team, and the composition of those teams varies widely: 87% contain an RN, 82% have a social worker, 77% have a physician, 65% have a chaplain, 41% have an advance practice nurse, 30% have a child life specialist, 32% have an integrative therapist, and 28% have a certified nursing assistant. What is also astonishing is that due to the vast shortage of pediatric-specific training of subspecialists, almost half (46%) of the organizations who responded to the NHPCO's Needs Assessment contract out roles (NHPCO, 2023).

Growth of services and the composition of these services has been a topic of much discussion and resulted in primary standards and recommendations from the AAP, the Center to Advance Palliative Care (CAPC), the Pediatric Palliative Care Quality Network, and NHPCO (Postier et al., 2024). These guidelines recommend including physicians, nurses, social workers, care managers, spiritual care providers, bereavement specialists, and child life specialists trained in pediatric palliative care. Despite the long-standing and harmonious recommendations of these organizations, teams continue to be variably composed and regularly understaffed. In some programs working to care for children, there may only be one team member (often a prescriber or social worker) trying to make up for a team's worth of professionals by themselves. As the field of pediatric palliative care evolves, developed or mature teams should follow the AAP's guidelines and expand into comprehensive PPC teams. In addition to having enough dedicated and trained staff to provide 24-7 pediatric palliative consultation, the care should be expanded beyond the inpatient arena and provide services in homes, schools, clinics, and participating facilities. PPC teams should also actively engage in research, ongoing quality improvement, and projects aimed at improving patient and family experiences and outcomes (AAP, 2013).

Inpatient work will always constitute a sizable portion of pediatric palliative care delivery, especially as the technology supporting children with serious illness advances. However, in the following section, we will look at how the focus of pediatric palliative care delivery is expanding to care for children outside the hospital's walls.

4.3   Outpatient Pediatric Palliative Care

Outpatient pediatric palliative care refers to a varied collection of services for children and families outside of the hospital. These offerings may include outpatient clinics, home-based programs, care in nonhospital facilities, and care through telehealth that reaches into the home. These programs have been developed in response to the perceived fragmentation of care between the hospital and home. The common thread in this diverse group of services is the intention to ensure that patients and families have what they need when they need it and where they prefer to receive it. Of the pediatric palliative programs evaluated in the United States in 2023, there were 48 eligible sites providing outpatient PPC. Of those 48 sites, 36 completed the survey and 28 clinics were identified. Top referral indications included pain management, goals of care, and advance care planning (Autrey et al., 2023). An important variation to note in the programs recently surveyed by Palliative Care Quality Collaborative is the composition of the teams who care for patients outside of the hospital (Weaver et al., 2023). The interdisciplinary team in the outpatient sphere is significantly decreased as often the patient will have a visit with a PPC physician, nurse practitioner or physician assistant, sometimes with a nurse and/or social worker, and rarely with a chaplain or child life specialist.

While some centers have practiced outpatient palliative care from their inception, growth of outpatient palliative care offerings has lagged in comparison to their inpatient counterparts. However, recent trends in serious illness care and health care in general have shown a renewed focus on allowing patients to stay in their preferred setting outside of the hospital. This has been bolstered by the ability for remote patient monitoring (Sasangohar et al., 2018), efficient workflows within durable medical equipment and home health services, and new patient service options that allow for quality clinical care in the home setting (Weaver et al., 2020, 2021; Boyden et al., 2021; Lin et al., 2020). The trajectory over the last several years suggests that outpatient palliative care is likely to grow more rapidly than inpatient palliative care in the future.

As outpatient PPC programs work to meet the needs of their community, they face challenges, including budget, staffing, and criteria for triaging involvement. Like their counterparts in the hospital, home-based programs cannot cover all their expenses through the reimbursement offered in the current system of private and public insurance. These programs rely on support from local health care organizations (affiliated and otherwise) along with philanthropic funds. These funds are very much appreciated, though reliance on outside funding puts programs at risk when economic or operational changes impact these partners. It is not uncommon for a high-quality, well-run program to encounter times of austerity or even close when such circumstances emerge. Data from outpatient clinics suggest programs can improve patient satisfaction, symptom control, and quality of life, and reduce health care utilization (Rabow et al., 2013, 2014); these benefits can help organizations justify their investment in outpatient programs. Unfortunately, without an aligned goal (financial or otherwise) this may be interesting and important data that fails to rally funds. As with all health care, especially pediatric subspecialties, palliative care faces a supply and demand imbalance in all its disciplines. This is compounded by a training pipeline with fewer training programs and trainees than can meet the needs of local and national communities (Dingfield et al., 2020). While this problem impacts all palliative care teams, outpatient work is hit especially hard due to the need for these caregivers to work more independently than many of their inpatient colleagues. This means that they need to have skill and mastery going into the job, rather than relying on a full team to mentor and develop their skills through direct observation in an inpatient setting.

Palliative care teams have approached the issue of staffing with creativity and collaboration. Some of the proposed solutions to this include community-based PPC services and home-based PPC teams as well as telehealth care services (Kaye et al., 2015). In a recent study, 46% of the outpatient clinics surveyed were able to provide separate home-based pediatric palliative care services in their area (Autrey et al., 2023). Home-based visits allow the provider to evaluate the patient in the patient's primary environment. In addition to the opportunity to get to know the patient and family more personally, home visits may reveal unseen obstacles to care and opportunities to enhance quality of life for the patient and their household (Weaver et al., 2020, 2021; Boyden et al., 2021; Lin et al., 2020).

Some distinct benefits of outpatient palliative care include the ability for families to plan and control the timing and agenda of these visits and improving interaction in discussing serious and emotionally charged topics. It also allows patients to be followed longitudinally for symptoms and needs, and for palliative care providers to connect with the teams that care for the patient outside of the hospital (Boyden et al., 2021). Inpatient palliative care teams often meet families at the height of stress when the limbic system, rather than higher level functioning, has taken over. Decisions may be made from a place of fear, anger, or hope in the heat of the moment. Working with families outside of these circumstances allows abstract thought and long-term perspective, which are extremely important when considering the complex plans for a child's future. Additionally, palliative care teams in hospitals are often actively involved in creating symptom management plans and do their best to design home regimens that will serve the child and family. Outpatient teams have an enhanced ability to see what life is like for patients outside of the hospital, which may be quite different from how they present in a hospital setting. This insight allows for safer and more effective prescribing and management of unique issues. It also may inform the goals that the patient and family are hoping for and the feasibility of accomplishing these goals. The primary care team for patients with serious illness is often expansive and not always visible to the inpatient team. Palliative care in the community may have a better working knowledge of the primary care team, homecare resources, nursing support, and other services that work for the good of a child. These working relationships bolster support for the patient, family, and the other professionals in the community. Many pediatric palliative care teams also co-visit with other subspecialists and/or participate in interdisciplinary meetings where patients are discussed. This collaboration magnifies the individual provider's ability to impact the care of a population of children.

Moving forward, outpatient pediatric palliative care will continue to grow and play a significant role in the care of children with serious illness. Our ability to leverage strategies such as community-based PPC services, home-based PPC teams, and telehealth care services will be closely related to our capacity to create and maintain structures that support this clear need and benefit children and their families.

4.4   Increasing Access to Pediatric Palliative Care Through Telehealth Services

The gold standard is providing access to care that meets patients where they are, both physically and existentially. Telehealth offers an opportunity to extend the reach of pediatric palliative care teams across the nation into health care deserts and rural and tribal communities. A form of tele-palliative care called remote patient monitoring was developed early in the 2010s and expanded rapidly in the context of the COVID-19 pandemic beginning in 2020. In a recent study, 75% of the outpatient clinics surveyed have telehealth access and the ability to conduct telehealth visits. Telehealth access has significantly expanded the range of pediatric palliative care teams while adding capabilities that may have been difficult to access for those visiting in person (Winegard et al., 2017; Weaver et al., 2021; Bradford et al., 2014). Access to language services is built into many telehealth platforms, allowing families in more remote areas to benefit from this essential service. Telehealth also provides a low-barrier opportunity for people in the child's care team to join a visit. This might include medical professionals, such as their primary care provider, or family members who play a key role but might otherwise be unable to join a clinic visit due to employment, illness, or geography. Many continue to prefer in-person interaction, though the benefits of telehealth in the outpatient setting ensure that it will be an important ingredient in any outpatient program.

In a systematic review in 2021 (Shah & Badawy) of randomized controlled trials that included telehealth for pediatric patients, telehealth was comparable to or better than in-person services. Although the studies focused on diseases like otitis media, skin conditions, mental health conditions, cystic fibrosis, and asthma, the outcomes measured in the study were related to symptom management, quality of life, satisfaction, medication adherence, visit completion rates, and disease progression (Shah & Badawy, 2021). Given these outcomes, it is possible that telehealth could be effectively used to overcome some of the barriers that exist for both inpatient and outpatient palliative care needs. It does not, however, replace the value of the face-to-face in-person encounter that is often highly beneficial to patients and their families when discussing serious illness, suffering, and the dynamic physical, emotional, spiritual, and existential impacts on life. This is well elucidated by Dr. Mehta (2021) in her article on remote patient monitoring in pediatric palliative care.

4.5 Barriers to Accessing Pediatric Palliative Care

4.5.1 Systemic Barriers

Systemic factors in the United States impact patient access to adequate pediatric palliative care. These include program funding, insurance coverage policies, staffing constraints, and lack of provider education.

Inconsistent and sometimes inadequate insurance coverage can limit access to pediatric palliative care. Coverage of PPC services varies across regions and socioeconomic status. Variability in state Medicaid programs and private insurance plans is an example of this inconsistency (Haines et al., 2018). If families need to move across state lines during treatment, care can be disrupted due to these variable coverage policies. Concurrent care hospice is only consistently available to patients with Medicaid insurance who are 21 years of age or younger, making this valuable resource sometimes out of reach for youth covered by private insurance.

An additional barrier to access to PPC is lack of program funding. Many hospitals are reluctant to allocate already strained financial resources to a program that tends to be revenue negative. In practice, there are strong arguments that PPC involvement improves resource utilization in pediatric hospitals. A retrospective study of 425 children with noncancer diagnoses receiving pediatric palliative care in the United States demonstrated a 38-day decrease in hospital length of stay and a savings of $275,000 per patient compared to resource utilization for those same patients prior to PPC enrollment (Postier et al., 2014).

Finally, there exists a nationwide shortage of clinicians with expertise in delivering palliative care, especially to children with cancer (Haines et al., 2018). Few residency and fellowship programs provide formal training in PPC, and pediatric oncologists are not typically trained in this area (Friedman et al., 2005). A 2021 survey of 54 PPC programs nationally identified that only 37% met minimum standards of practice for staffing (Rogers et al., 2021). Even for large hospitals with robust PPC programs, staffing constraints often limit the number of patients they can support.

4.5.2 Access Disparities Based on Social Identity

Disparities in access to palliative care based on race, ethnicity, language preference, and cultural identities have been well documented in the adult literature. These studies show that BIPOC, LGBTQ, and disabled populations are less likely to use hospice, have lower satisfaction with care, receive care that is less aligned with their preferences, and have decreased access to medications (Marcewicz et al., 2022; Haviland et al., 2021; Velepucha-Iniguez et al., 2022; Patel et al., 2023). While these disparities have been less well explored in the pediatric population, we know that racism and discrimination based on language preference exist in our hospitals

(Purtell et al., 2021). For example, Hispanic families of children with cancer report receiving care that is less aligned with their goals at the end of life compared to white families (Kaye et al., 2019). In a study of 426 children with cancer, white patients spent fewer days in the hospital in the last 3 months of life compared to Black, Asian, and Hispanic patients (DeGroote et al., 2022).

Cultural beliefs and identities can impact how families prefer to engage with palliative care teams. They influence whether the family values the involvement of clergy, how they wish to receive information (e.g., direct versus indirect communication), how nonverbal cues are interpreted, how they wish to talk about death and dying with children, their understanding of the meaning of pain and suffering, their beliefs regarding the meaning of death and dying, and their preferred location for end-of-life care (Wiener et al., 2013). Lack of awareness of these nuances can damage trust and rapport (Cain et al., 2018). Different institutions have different levels of education and experience regarding cultural humility, awareness of social identities, and rigor of data tracking discrimination/bias safety events, all of which can impact the frequency with which these communication breakdowns occur (McKee et al., 2022).

4.5.3 Perceptions Toward Palliative Care

Family preferences not being aligned with palliative care are often cited in the literature as barriers to PPC involvement. In a mixed-methods study among pediatric trainees and faculty physicians at three pediatric hospitals, perceptions of barriers to PPC involvement included family not being ready to acknowledge an incurable condition, family preference for more life-sustaining therapies, uncertain prognosis, and parent discomfort with the possibility of hastening death (Levine et al., 2023). These perceptions can represent a gap in understanding of the function and value of PPC as none of these preferences are contraindications to palliative involvement. In fact, prognostic uncertainty should be a sign to initiate rather than delay a palliative care consult, and many families can receive holistic palliative support while continuing to pursue cure and without hastening death (Davies et al., 2008). In fact, both adult and pediatric data suggest that hospice involvement prolongs life expectancy at a higher quality of life (Eichelberger & Shadiack, 2018; Friedrichsdorf, 2010).

Provider perceptions of PPC may also demonstrate a gap in understanding the value of PPC involvement and act as a barrier to its utilization. Much of PPC is provided as an inpatient consultative service, meaning providers must make a referral to the PPC team. Here, a lack of provider awareness of and willingness to discuss PPC with patients and families can act as a barrier to PPC involvement (Haines et al., 2018). A lack of education and training specific to PPC among pediatric providers can lead to misunderstandings regarding the purpose and value of PPC, resulting in barriers to its utilization (Haines et al., 2018; Balkin et al., 2017; Davies et al., 2008). Such misconceptions include the beliefs that palliative care is synonymous with hospice or end-of-life care, that palliative care cannot be delivered alongside curative treatments, and that pediatric patients are unable to participate in discussions regarding palliative care (Haines et al., 2018). Research also indicates that providers perceive PPC consultations as helpful but occurring "too late" (Balkin et al., 2017; Afonso et al., 2021).

In a survey of 183 pediatric cardiologists and cardiac surgeons regarding attitudes toward PPC, researchers identified the following perceived barriers to requesting PPC consultation: concern that consultation occurring too early will undermine hope and concern that consultation will be perceived by the patient's family as "giving up" (Balkin et al., 2017). Additional provider-perceived barriers to the utilization of PPC include prognostic uncertainty, language barriers, time constraints, and family not being ready to acknowledge an incurable condition (Davies et al., 2008; Levine et al., 2023). Provider personal beliefs may also serve as barriers to PPC consultation. For example, discomfort in initiating conversations about PPC can hinder consultation (Haines et al., 2018). Conflict between staff and family regarding treatment goals (e.g., family preference for more life-sustaining therapies than staff) is also cited as a barrier to PPC consultation (Davies et al., 2008; Levine et al., 2023).

These findings highlight the need for education about the scope of practice of palliative care and training to increase understanding and clarify misconceptions.

References

Afonso, N. S., Ninemire, M. R., Gowda, S. H., Jump, J. L., Lantin-Hermoso, R. L., Johnson, K. E., Puri, K., Hope, K. D., Kritz, E., Achuff, B. J., Gurganious, L., & Bhat, P. N. (2021). Redefining the relationship: Palliative care in critical perinatal and neonatal cardiac patients. *Children (Basel), 8*(7), 548. https://doi.org/10.3390/children8070548

American Academy of Pediatrics (AAP), Section on Hospice and Palliative Medicine and Committee on Hospital Care. (2013). Pediatric palliative care and hospice care commitments, guidelines, and recommendations. *Pediatrics, 132*(5), 966–972. https://doi.org/10.1542/peds.2013-2731

Autrey, A. K., James, C., Sarvode Mothi, S., Stafford, C., Morvant, A., Miller, E. G., & Kaye, E. C. (2023). The landscape of outpatient pediatric palliative care: A national cross-sectional assessment. *Journal of Pain and Symptom Management, 66*(1), 1–23. https://doi.org/10.1016/j.jpainsymman.2023.02.006

Balkin, E. M., Kirkpatrick, J. N., Kaufman, B., Swetz, K. M., Sleeper, L. A., Wolfe, J., & Blume, E. D. (2017). Pediatric cardiology provider attitudes about palliative care: A multicenter survey study. *Pediatric Cardiology, 38*(7), 1324–1331. https://doi.org/10.1007/s00246-017-1663-0

Bergstraesser, E. (2013). Pediatric palliative care-when quality of life becomes the main focus of treatment. *European Journal of Pediatrics, 172*(2), 139–150. https://doi.org/10.1007/s00431-012-1710-z

Boyden, J. Y., Ersek, M., Deatrick, J. A., Widger, K., LaRagione, G., Lord, B., & Feudtner, C. (2021). What do parents value regarding pediatric palliative and hospice care in the home setting? *Journal of Pain and Symptom Management, 61*(1), 12–23. https://doi.org/10.1016/j.jpainsymman.2020.07.024

Bradford, N. K., Armfield, N. R., Young, J., Herbert, A., Mott, C., & Smith, A. C. (2014). Principles of a paediatric palliative care consultation can be achieved with home telemedicine. *Journal of Telemedicine and Telecare, 20*(7), 360–364. https://doi.org/10.1177/1357633X14552370

Cain, C. L., Surbone, A., Elk, R., & Kagawa-Singer, M. (2018). Culture and palliative care: Preferences, communication, meaning, and mutual decision making. *Journal of Pain and Symptom Management, 55*(5), 1408–1419. https://doi.org/10.1016/j.jpainsymman.2018.01.007

Davies, B., Sehring, S. A., Partridge, J. C., Cooper, B. A., Hughes, A., Philp, J. C., Amidi-Nouri, A., & Kramer, R. F. (2008). Barriers to palliative care for children: Perceptions of pediatric health care providers. *Pediatrics, 121*(2), 282–288. https://doi.org/10.1542/peds.2006-3153

DeGroote, N. P., Allen, K. E., Falk, E. E., Velozzi-Averhoff, C., Wasilewski-Masker, K., Johnson, K., & Brock, K. E. (2022). Relationship of race and ethnicity on access, timing, and disparities in pediatric palliative care for children with cancer. *Supportive Care in Cancer, 30*(1), 923–930. https://doi.org/10.1007/s00520-021-06500-6

Dingfield, L. E., Jackson, V. A., deLima Thomas, J., Doyle, K. P., Ferris, F., & Radwany, S. M. (2020). Looking back, and ahead: A call to action for increasing the hospice and palliative medicine specialty pipeline. *Journal of Palliative Medicine, 23*(7), 895–899. https://doi.org/10.1089/jpm.2020.0008

Eichelberger, T., & Shadiack, A. (2018). Life expectancy with hospice care. *American Family Physician, 97*(5). Retrieved from https://www.aafp.org/pubs/afp/issues/2018/0301/od2.html

Feudtner, C., Womer, J., Augustin, R., Remke, S., Wolfe, J., Friebert, S., & Weissman, D. (2013). Pediatric palliative care programs in children's hospitals: A cross-sectional national survey. *Pediatrics, 132*(6), 1063–1070. https://doi.org/10.1542/peds.2013-1286

Friedman, D. L., Hilden, J. M., & Powaski, K. (2005). Issues and challenges in palliative care for children with cancer. *Current Pain and Headache Reports, 9*(4), 249–255. https://doi.org/10.1007/s11916-005-0032-5

Friedrichsdorf, S. J. (2010). Pain management in children with advanced cancer and during end-of-life care. *Pediatric Hematology and Oncology, 27*(4), 257–261. https://doi.org/10.3109/08880011003663416

Haines, E. R., Frost, A. C., Kane, H. L., & Rokoske, F. S. (2018). Barriers to accessing palliative care for pediatric patients with cancer: A review of the literature. *Cancer, 124*(11), 2278–2288. https://doi.org/10.1002/cncr.31265

Haviland, K., Burrows Walters, C., & Newman, S. (2021). Barriers to palliative care in sexual and gender minority patients with cancer: A scoping review of the literature. *Health & Social Care in the Community, 29*(2), 305–318. https://doi.org/10.1111/hsc.13126

Kaye, E. C., Rubenstein, J., Levine, D., Baker, J. N., Dabbs, D., & Friebert, S. E. (2015). Pediatric palliative care in the community. *CA: A Cancer Journal for Clinicians, 65*(4), 316–333. https://doi.org/10.3322/caac.21280

Kaye, E. C., Gushue, C. A., DeMarsh, S., Jerkins, J., Li, C., Lu, Z., Snaman, J. M., Blazin, L., Johnson, L. M., Levine, D. R., Morrison, R. R., & Baker, J. N. (2019). Impact of race and ethnicity on end-of-life experiences for children with cancer. *American Journal of Hospice & Palliative Care, 36*(9), 767–774. https://doi.org/10.1177/1049909119836939

Keele, L., Keenan, H. T., & Bratton, S. L. (2016). The effect of palliative care team design on referrals to pediatric palliative care. *Journal of Palliative Medicine, 19*(3), 286–291. https://doi.org/10.1089/jpm.2015.0261

Levine, A., Winn, P. A., Fogel, A. H., Lelkes, E., McPoland, P., Agrawal, A. K., & Bogetz, J. F. (2023). Barriers to pediatric palliative care: Trainee and faculty perspectives across two academic centers. *Journal of Palliative Medicine, 26*(10), 1348–1356. https://doi.org/10.1089/jpm.2022.0580

Lin, E., Scharbach, K., Liu, B., Braun, M., Tannis, C., Wilson, K., & Truglio, J. (2020). A multidisciplinary home visiting program for children with medical complexity. *Hospital Pediatrics, 10*(11), 925–931. https://doi.org/10.1542/hpeds.2020-0093

Marcewicz, L., Kunihiro, S. K., Curseen, K. A., Johnson, K., & Kavalieratos, D. (2022). Application of critical race theory in palliative care research: A scoping review. *Journal of Pain and Symptom Management, 63*(6), e667–e684. https://doi.org/10.1016/j.jpainsymman.2022.02.018

McKee, M. N., Palama, B. K., Hall, M., LaBelle, J. L., Bohr, N. L., & Hoehn, K. S. (2022). Racial and ethnic differences in inpatient palliative care for pediatric stem cell transplant patients. *Pediatric Critical Care Medicine, 23*(6), 417–424. https://doi.org/10.1097/PCC.0000000000002916

Mehta, A. (2021). Remote patient monitoring in pediatric palliative/hospice care: A physician's perspective. In C. Corr (Ed.), *NHPCO pediatric E-journal issue #63* (pp. 17–20). Pediatric Advisory Council. https://www.nhpco.org/wp-content/uploads/ChiPPS_E-Journal_Issue_63.pdf

National Hospice and Palliative Care Organization (NHPCO). (2023). *NHPCO pediatric facts and figures* (23rd ed.). National Hospice and Palliative Care Organization. https://www.nhpco.org/wp-content/uploads/NHPCO_Pediatric_Facts_Figures_2023.pdf

Norris, S., Minkowitz, S., & Scharbach, K. (2019). Pediatric palliative care. *Primary Care, 46*(3), 461–473. https://doi.org/10.1016/j.pop.2019.05.010

Patel, R., Patel, D., Patel, Z., Patel, M., Chitkara, A., Yang, C., Onyechi, A., & Patel, F. (2023). Disparities in palliative care utilization in deceased lymphoma patients: A nationwide analysis, Abstract 131. *Blood, 142*(Supl 1), 131. https://doi.org/10.1182/blood-2023-174177

Postier, A., Chrastek, J., Nugent, S., Osenga, K., & Friedrichsdorf, S. J. (2014). Exposure to home-based pediatric palliative and hospice care and its impact on hospital and emergency care charges at a single institution. *Journal of Palliative Medicine, 17*(2), 183–188. https://doi.org/10.1089/jpm.2013.0287

Postier, A. C., Root, M. C., O'Riordan, D. L., Purser, L., Friedrichsdorf, S. J., Pantilat, S. Z., & Bogetz, J. F. (2024). The pediatric palliative care quality network: Palliative care consultation and patient outcomes. *Hospital Pediatrics, 14*(1), 1–10. https://doi.org/10.1542/hpeds.2023-007222

Purtell, R., Tam, R. P., Avondet, E., & Gradick, K. (2021). We are part of the problem: The role of children's hospitals in addressing health inequity. *Hospital Practice, 49*(Supl), 445–455. https://doi.org/10.1080/21548331.2022.2032072

Rabow, M., Kvale, E., Barbour, L., Cassel, J. B., Cohen, S., Jackson, V., Luhrs, C., Nguyen, V., Rinaldi, S., Stevens, D., Spragens, L., & Weissman, D. (2013). Moving upstream: A review of the evidence of the impact of outpatient palliative care. *Journal of Palliative Medicine, 16*(12), 1540–1549. https://doi.org/10.1089/jpm.2013.0153

Rabow, M. W., O'Riordan, D. L., & Pantilat, S. Z. (2014). A statewide survey of adult and pediatric outpatient palliative care services. *Journal of Palliative Medicine, 17*(12), 1311–1316. https://doi.org/10.1089/jpm.2014.0144

Rogers, M., & Kirch, R. (2019, May 15). *Spotlight on pediatric palliative care: National Landscape of Hospital-Based Programs, 2015–16*. Center to Advance Palliative Care. Retrieved February 15, 2024, from https://www.capc.org/blog/palliative-pulse-palliative-pulse-july-2017-spotlight-pediatric-palliative-care-national-landscape-hospital-based-programs-2015-2016/

Rogers, M. M., Friebert, S., Williams, C. S. P., Humphrey, L., Thienprayoon, R., & Klick, J. C. (2021). Pediatric palliative care programs in US hospitals. *Pediatrics, 148*(1), e2020021634. https://doi.org/10.1542/peds.2020-021634

Sasangohar, F., Davis, E., Kash, B. A., & Shah, S. R. (2018). Remote patient monitoring and telemedicine in neonatal and pediatric settings: Scoping literature review. *Journal of Medical Internet Research, 20*(12), e295. https://doi.org/10.2196/jmir.9403

Shah, A. C., & Badawy, S. M. (2021). Telemedicine in pediatrics: Systematic review of randomized controlled trials. *JMIR Pediatrics and Parenting, 4*(1), e22696. https://doi.org/10.2196/22696

Sisk, B. A., Feudtner, C., Bluebond-Langner, M., Sourkes, B., Hinds, P. S., & Wolfe, J. (2020). Response to suffering of the seriously ill child: A history of palliative care for children. *Pediatrics, 145*(1), e20191741. https://doi.org/10.1542/peds.2019-1741

Srinivasan, V. J., Akhtar, S., Huppertz, J. W., Sidhu, M., Coates, A., & Knudsen, N. (2023). Prospective cohort study on the impact of early versus late inpatient palliative care on length of stay and cost of care. *The American Journal of Hospice & Palliative Care, 40*(7), 704–710. https://doi.org/10.1177/10499091231152609

Velepucha-Iniguez, J., Bonilla Sierra, P., & Bruera, E. (2022). Barriers to palliative care access in patients with intellectual disability: A scoping review. *Journal of Pain and Symptom Management, 64*(6), e347–e356. https://doi.org/10.1016/j.jpainsymman.2022.08.007

Weaver, M. S., Rosenberg, A. R., Tager, J., Wichman, C. S., & Wiener, L. (2018). A summary of pediatric palliative care team structure and services as reported by centers caring for children with cancer. *Journal of Palliative Medicine, 21*(4), 452–462. https://doi.org/10.1089/jpm.2017.0405

Weaver, M. S., Robinson, J. E., Shostrom, V. K., & Hinds, P. S. (2020). Telehealth acceptability for children, family, and adult hospice nurses when integrating the pediatric palliative inpatient provider during sequential rural home hospice visits. *Journal of Palliative Medicine, 23*(5), 641–649. https://doi.org/10.1089/jpm.2019.0450

Weaver, M. S., Shostrom, V. K., Neumann, M. L., Robinson, J. E., & Hinds, P. S. (2021). Homestead together: Pediatric palliative care telehealth support for rural children with cancer during home-based end-of-life care. *Pediatric Blood & Cancer, 68*(4), e28921. https://doi.org/10.1002/pbc.28921

Weaver, M. S., Shostrom, V. K., Kaye, E. C., Keegan, A., & Lindley, L. C. (2022). Palliative care programs in children's hospitals. *Pediatrics, 150*(4), e2022057872. https://doi.org/10.1542/peds.2022-057872

Weaver, M. S., Chana, T., Fisher, D., Fost, H., Hawley, B., James, K., Lindley, L. C., Samson, K., Smith, S. M., Ware, A., & Torkildson, C. (2023). State of the service: Pediatric palliative and hospice community-based service coverage in the United States. *Journal of Palliative Medicine, 26*(11), 1521–1528. https://doi.org/10.1089/jpm.2023.0204

Wiener, L., McConnell, D. G., Latella, L., & Ludi, E. (2013). Cultural and religious considerations in pediatric palliative care. *Palliative & Supportive Care, 11*(1), 47–67. https://doi.org/10.1017/S1478951511001027

Winegard, B., Miller, E. G., & Slamon, N. B. (2017). Use of telehealth in pediatric palliative care. *Telemedicine Journal and E-Health, 23*(11), 938–940. https://doi.org/10.1089/tmj.2016.0251

Chapter 5
The Future of Pediatric Palliative Care

5.1 Expanding Pediatric Palliative Care by National Organization Endorsement

A variety of national and international organizations endorse pediatric palliative care (PPC) and its value in the health care system. The guidelines and recommendations for PPC and pediatric hospice care (PHC) put forth by the American Academy of Pediatrics (AAP, 2013) include ensuring that all hospitals and large health care organizations that routinely serve children with life-threatening conditions have dedicated interdisciplinary PPC-PHC teams; that PPC-PHC competencies be included in medical school, residency, and fellowship curricula; that PPC-PHC teams support ongoing research and quality improvement; and that PPC-PHC be paid equitably across settings to ensure access to high-quality care for patients and families. In its clinical report on guidance for pediatric end-of-life care, the AAP supports early engagement of palliative care and advocacy to expand its availability in both hospital and community settings (Linebarger et al., 2022). Many of these aspects of PPC are evident in the initial statement on palliative care for children put forth by the AAP in 2000. Here, the following principles were outlined as foundational to an integrated model of palliative care: respect for the dignity of patients and families, both during their illness and after the child's death; access to competent and compassionate palliative care in order to improve quality of life; support for health care professionals to process the emotions associated with caring for the dying child; improved support for pediatric palliative care through education; and continued improvement of pediatric palliative care through research, education, and practice (AAP, 2000).

In a recent statement, the American Heart Association emphasized the importance of palliative care involvement for children with heart disease due to morbidity and mortality risks, stating that "the clinical course for patients with complex

C. Delgado-Corcoran et al., *Specialized Pediatric Palliative Care*,
SpringerBriefs in Public Health, https://doi.org/10.1007/978-3-031-65452-7_5

congenital [heart disease] and pediatric acquired [heart disease] with potential for future heart failure necessitates early and longitudinal primary palliative care" (Blume et al., 2023, p. 175). The statement further details that pediatric cardiology and cardiovascular surgery trainees should receive relevant training on palliative care skills and utilize them within their scope of practice (Blume et al., 2023).

In their clinical training recommendations for all clinicians caring for pediatric patients, including physicians, physician assistants, advanced practice registered nurses, registered nurses, and social workers, the Center to Advance Palliative Care (n.d.) identifies as a necessary skill the ability to identify those patients who would benefit from a specialty pediatric palliative care consultation to assist with symptom management for complex or intractable symptoms.

In the clinical practice guidelines for quality palliative care published by the National Coalition for Hospice and Palliative Care (National Consensus Project for Quality Palliative Care, 2018) and endorsed by the American Academy of Pediatrics (2019), several pertinent recommendations are made: to provide the highest quality care that meets the holistic needs of patients and families, palliative care should be provided by an interdisciplinary team with training in palliative care; this commitment to optimal patient- and family-centered care catered to the unique physical, psychological, and spiritual needs of each patient and family should be evident in assessment, care planning, and treatment (National Consensus Project for Quality Palliative Care, 2018).

The World Health Organization (WHO) recognizes palliative care as being promotive of better patient outcomes including improved pain control, health-related quality of life, family satisfaction, and emotional well-being in addition to reduced health care costs. In their guide for integrating palliative care and symptom relief into pediatrics, palliative care is described as "… an essential complement to curative or disease-modifying treatments for serious or life-threatening health condition" (WHO, 2018, p. 51).

5.2   Pediatric Palliative Care Research: Resources and Expansion

5.2.1   Addressing Research Challenges in Pediatric Palliative Care

Researchers in palliative care face significant obstacles to conducting high-quality research despite the identification of gaps in knowledge partly due to lack of funding, limited research workforce, and challenges related to public and professional misunderstanding of palliative care (Chen et al., 2014). Pediatric palliative care researchers are challenged by the use of small and heterogeneous study populations experiencing rapid changes in health status (Beecham et al., 2016). Referral patterns to PPC services and research participant representation demonstrate unfair patterns.

For example, young people who are African American, live in rural or low-income areas, or do not have private insurance are referred less frequently (Nelson et al., 2018). The overwhelming majority of pediatric palliative care study participants are white, and many studies limit participation to English-speaking families (Sample et al., 2021). Participating family members are typically white mothers, limiting input from other family members (Nelson et al., 2018). Addressing these inequities through use of referral triggers, analysis of demographic information, and intentional study design can make research findings more equitable and applicable to all who may benefit (Nelson et al., 2018; Mooney-Doyle et al., 2022).

In a systematic review of the impact of specialized palliative care by Marcus et al. (2020), over half of the studies exhibited participant selection bias given observational, retrospective structure and low survey response rates with lack of comparisons between responders and nonresponders. Thus, there is ample opportunity for future studies utilizing validated tools and specific standardized outcomes in controlled settings.

Study designs have rarely represented the voices of young people receiving care, relying heavily or completely on often discordant proxy reporting (Friedel et al., 2019). Challenges to their participation include communication and ethics of assent. Assent processes require attention as parental decision-making and assent of children are viewed differently across cultural contexts (Khoo et al., 2023). Further, children with life-limiting illnesses have varied abilities to comprehend considerations or communicate preferences. Strategies such as questions that are read aloud or use of communication devices allow children to complete surveys despite physical or cognitive barriers (Nelson et al., 2018). Diversity of ages among participants experiencing illness is also important, particularly since certain age groups are known to have poorer psychosocial outcomes (Lau et al., 2020).

Despite early and ongoing concerns about traumatizing participants, surveys of families engaged in pediatric palliative care research have shown that benefits outweigh burdens (Weaver et al., 2019). Families found meaning in opportunities to help others, reflect on and share their stories, and remember their children (Hasan et al., 2021).

Challenges of doing palliative care research may be ameliorated by standardized measures, the use of diverse populations, input from young people and caregivers, and utilizing communication support when needed (Nelson et al., 2018).

5.2.2 Research Resources and Methodologies

Creative study design, cooperative research resources, use of databases, increased numbers of practitioners, development of validated tools, and increased funding have supported the growth of palliative care research. During the last 5 years, researchers have contributed numerous multisite, prospective, and randomized control trials.

5.2.2.1 Databases

Grouped information, through multisite studies or database utilization, has resulted in increased sample size and study rigor in PPC (Visser et al., 2015). Database resources include the Pediatric Palliative Care Research Network's SHAred Data and REsearch (SHARE), an interdisciplinary effort of six children's hospitals. Family demographics, goals of care, psychological health, and symptom priorities are recorded. Patient-related information such as prescriptions, diagnoses, procedures, and symptom data is also collected (Nye et al., 2022).

The Palliative Care Research Cooperative (PCRC) supports palliative care research for adult and pediatric populations. Similar to SHARE, it offers support for multidisciplinary researchers as well as a repository (Ritchie et al., 2017). First funded by the National Institute for Nursing Research, PCRC was created to support high-quality palliative care research, with emphasis on multisite and new investigator processes.

The Children's Hospital Association manages the Pediatric Health Information System (PHIS) database, which includes information about young people who receive care at 49 US children's hospitals. Encounters for surgery, emergency department, observation, inpatient, and ambulatory care are recorded. Demographic, procedure, and billing data are associated with each encounter (Children's Hospital Association, n.d.).

The Patient-reported Outcome Measurement Information System (PROMIS) (Health Measures, 2023), initiated with the National Institutes of Health funding in 2004, offers resources for self-reporting of patients' physical, social, mental, and global health. Resources are available electronically and on paper, with some tools in English and Spanish.

5.2.2.2 Tool Selection

Two tools have been used to assess the eligibility for PPC and facilitate timely and appropriate PPC referral of children between 1 and 18 years old. One is the Pediatric Palliative Screening Scale (PaPaS) and the other is the Assessment Form for Complex Clinical Needs in Pediatrics (ACCAPED) Scale (Papa et al., 2023). The PaPaS scale assesses the care burden of the child and caregivers, while the ACCAPED scale assesses the clinical needs of a child with a life-limiting or life-threatening illness. Both scales specify whether a family would be well served by generalist palliative care or whether specialty care is necessary (Papa et al., 2023).

Regarding the measurement of family needs, general tools that have been validated in the pediatric palliative care population include the Pediatric Palliative Care Early Intervention Tool, a nurse-driven instrument that quantifies patient symptom needs; the Family Empowerment Scale, which measures parental sense of control; and PCNeeds, which includes relationship and decision-making needs (Papa et al., 2023). Tools for evaluation of specific symptoms (e.g., pain, sleep quality, nausea) are available for PPC patients but have not yet been validated. A more comprehensive list of specific tools designed to evaluate symptoms are found in articles by Pinheiro et al. in 2018 and Chan et al. in 2022.

Measurement of palliative care treatment efficacy and quality of life can be performed using care assessment tools like the African Children's Palliative Outcome Scale (C-POS) as a brief assessment (Papa et al., 2023). The FACETS-OF-PPC, a lengthier tool, is useful for young people with severe neurological impairment (Papa et al., 2023). Other assessment tools noted in the literature include the Hospital Anxiety and Depression Scale (HADS), the Pediatric Quality of Life (Peds QL) 4.0, the Supportive Care sCore (SCC), the Quality of Life in Life-Threatening Illness-Family Caregiver Questionnaire (QOLLTI-F), and the Needs at the End of Life (NEST) screening tool (Friedel et al., 2019). Additional tools await validation for broader use.

Lastly, retrospective evaluation of parents' experiences related to their child's end of life can be evaluated using the Parental PELICAN questionnaire. The tool is setting-specific, with versions for neurology, cardiology, neonatology, and oncology (Papa et al., 2023).

5.2.2.3 Outcome Measures

The measures of morbidity and mortality common in other studies are less helpful in palliative care research as participants are known to have incurable illness and decreased life expectancy (Visser et al., 2015; Feudtner et al., 2019). Alternatively, researchers have utilized measures of quality of life, coping and stress, and symptom burden as outcome measures. Unfortunately, these outcomes measures are subjective, vary between child and parents, and are dependent on child age, duration of symptoms, and frequency of assessment, posing further research challenges in PPC (Feudtner et al., 2019).

5.2.2.4 Study Design

Challenges associated with population heterogeneity can be addressed through study design. Exposure-crossover design compares the rate of an outcome before and after a patient undergoes an exposure. Thus, patients are compared to themselves (Nelson et al., 2018). Latent class analysis can also be effective as it subdivides a larger population into groups of participants with multiple commonalities. These groups can then be compared to one another as outcomes are evaluated (Nelson et al., 2018). Longitudinal studies may be better for examining long-term outcomes and allowing for comparison of patients' disease trajectories and associated factors (Nelson et al., 2018; Visser et al., 2015). However, these studies are prone to missing data as PPC patients have a high level of morbidity and mortality, and are thus often unable to complete assessments, especially as their illness advances or their symptoms worsen (Nelson et al., 2018). Additionally, there are no standards for when reassessments should occur in longitudinal studies, limiting comparison across studies (Feudtner et al., 2019).

5.2.2.4.1   Randomized Clinical Trials Related to Pediatric Palliative Care

One example of a randomized clinical trial related to palliative care is the Family-Centered Advance Care Planning for Teens with Cancer (FACE-TC) study. The study was conducted from 2016 to 2019 at four children's hospitals to evaluate the longitudinal efficacy of the FACE-TC intervention to sustain adolescent–family congruence about end-of-life treatment preferences (Needle et al., 2022). The study enrolled adolescents (aged 14–21 years) with cancer and their family members for staged advance care planning discussions. A total of 126 adolescent–family dyads were randomized 2:1 to FACE-TC (intervention group $n = 83$) or treatment as usual (control group $n = 43$) and underwent five follow-up visits over an 18-month post-intervention period. Intention-to-treat analyses were conducted from March 2021 to April 2022 (Needle et al., 2022). The results of this trial showed that, for those who received the FACE-TC intervention, the families' knowledge of their adolescents' end-of-life treatment preferences was sustained for 1 year (Needle et al., 2022). The 126 dyads also completed the Functional Assessment of Chronic Illness Therapy-Spiritual Well-Being (FACIT-SP) Version 4 to evaluate congruence of family beliefs around treatment and spirituality (Livingston et al., 2020). Analysis of study data revealed that adolescents with cancer and their family members tended to share relational sentiments, such as compassion for others and feeling loved, but differed in concordance of religious sentiments (Livingston et al., 2020).

Another randomized trial is the Promoting Resilience in Stress Management (PRISM) study, conducted from January 2015 to October 2016, in which adolescents and young adults (12–25 years old) with cancer ($n = 92$) were randomized one-to-one to PRISM ($n = 48$) or usual care ($n = 44$). PRISM teaches stress management, goal setting, cognitive-reframing, and meaning-making skills. The intervention included four individual sessions of skill-building with optional monthly follow-up sessions. Outcome measures included hope, benefit-finding, general quality of life, distress, and cancer-specific quality of life. Participants completed surveys at enrollment and 6 months later. Researchers found that receiving PRISM was associated with improved benefit-finding and hope with clinically meaningful effect sizes when compared to usual care (Rosenberg et al., 2019).

As a part of the PRISM study, Seattle researchers conducted further analyses and examined whether response to PRISM differed across key sociodemographic characteristics (Lau et al., 2020). Participants were stratified by sex, age, race, and neighborhood socioeconomic disadvantage based on home address. The PRISM intervention demonstrated a positive effect for the majority of outcomes regardless of sex, age, and race, though it may not be as helpful for adolescents and young adults living in disadvantaged neighborhoods (Lau et al., 2020).

Similar interventions were offered to parents of young people with cancer in an associated PRISM study, with benefits shown after 3 months (Rosenberg et al.,

2019). Significant findings included increased resilience and benefit-finding in parents receiving 1:1 training. A follow-up publication described parental stress 6 months after baseline assessments (Rosenberg et al., 2021). Participants were randomized to usual care, or usual care with either 1:1 support or group PRISM education, with most participants being white, college-educated, English-speaking mothers. Both intervention groups received four sessions of skill-building instruction. Resilience, benefit-finding, and distress levels were measured at 3 and 6 months. The study showed benefits 3 months after the intervention but none at 6 months. Interestingly, findings showed that distress levels decreased over time even for the usual care group. Parents reported the training was helpful, particularly stress management teachings (Rosenberg et al., 2021).

A 2022 publication evaluated the findings of a randomized control trial regarding the early integration of palliative support for young people hospitalized for more than 8 days in a pediatric intensive care setting (Erçin-Swearinger et al., 2022). Outcome measures included prevalence of symptoms correlated with acute or post-traumatic stress disorders. English- and Spanish-speaking family members were included, with 377 family members and 220 children participating. Baseline measurements showed no significant differences in symptom prevalence. The study also examined family functioning, perceived support, and trust in medical providers. Analyses showed longer length of stay, lower family functioning, child's death, being a parent, and female gender were risk factors for manifestation of stress symptoms (Erçin-Swearinger et al., 2022). Among family members whose children died, over 41% met diagnostic criteria for post-traumatic stress disorder (PTSD); 9.7% of family members of children who did not die met these criteria. Over 15% of family members surveyed met the criteria for acute stress disorder. At 3-month follow-up, 13.8% of family members met the PTSD criteria. This study provides insight into the factors predisposing families to difficult courses. However, the study does not provide information regarding comparison between groups receiving palliative services and those in the control.

The Pediatric Quality of Life and Evaluation of Symptoms Technology (PediQUEST) trial, conducted between 2004 and 2009, was a three-site randomized control trial. Children with advanced cancer and their caregivers received palliative care support and regular self-report assessments (Wolfe et al., 2014). For each participating child with advanced cancer, the child or caregiver completed assessments weekly for 20 weeks. Assessments included the Memorial Symptom Assessment Scale and the Pediatric Quality of Life Inventory 4.0 (Peds QL4.0). There was also a question regarding general feeling of sickness. Child, parent, and provider satisfaction were also evaluated. Findings included significant improvement in Peds QL4.0 emotional scores and general sickness reports. Oncologists shared that reports yielded little helpful information regarding physical symptoms but did provide new information about psychosocial needs. Information did not tend to change oncologists' views about goals but did contribute to decisions to refer for social work, pain team, palliative care, or psychosocial support (Wolfe et al., 2014). A PediQUEST follow-up study assessed parent and child perspectives regarding patient-reported outcome report systems related to symptoms and quality of life

(Merz et al., 2023). Families noted that participation increased awareness regarding their own and others' experiences. They also reported improved communication among family members and care teams. The study used questions read aloud for children 5–8 years of age, and young people over 8 years completed their own reports. English- and Spanish-speaking families participated.

The PediQUEST Response study is a five-site randomized, controlled effectiveness trial conducted from March 2018 to September 2022 (Dussel et al., 2022). The updated web-based assessment tools are accessible by app for weekly completion by patients or family members. A primary goal is to improve health-related quality of life scores; secondary outcomes include implementation of treatment for symptoms and decreased stress and anxiety. Tools include the PediQUEST Memorial Symptom Assessment Scale, Spielberger's-State-Trait Anxiety Inventory, the Center for Epidemiologic Studies Short Depression Scale, and a pain-related portion of the Response to Stress Questionnaires (Dussel et al., 2022).

Other notable studies with randomized control designs have evaluated interventions addressing caregiver support for families with children in intensive care settings. One two-site study entailed a collection of supports to assist with decision-making, communication, informational, or end-of-life needs. Supports included a trained navigator, diary, question prompt list, bedside communication log, and information about the ICU including therapies administered (Michelson et al., 2020). Outcome measures included "excellent" responses to decision-making domains of family satisfaction surveys completed 3–5 weeks after discharge, as well as parental morbidities and perceptions of team communication. Navigators were masters-level professionals in social work, child development, family studies, or marriage and family therapy. Sample size was 382 families. While the service was rated positively by parents, there was no statistically significant difference in decision-making satisfaction, which researchers noted could be related to the underpowered study. Researchers did observe a shorter length of stay and smaller number of family meetings among the intervention group. The authors noted that multiple factors may have influenced study outcomes, including limited availability of navigators and family members, baseline parent characteristics, and indirect influence of care received by families in the nonintervention arm. Response bias was also noted as a disproportionate number of survey responses were from non-Hispanic white, educated parents (Michelson et al., 2020).

5.2.3 Future of Research in Pediatric Palliative Care

There is a need for adequately powered multisite studies with diverse participant groups, use of validated tools, effective and clear interventions, and clear desired outcomes. Fortunately, barriers are addressed through growing workforce, increased cooperation and support, and improved understanding of how research can benefit participating families.

5.3 Pediatric Palliative Care Education and Training Opportunities

The field of palliative care has seen significant expansion since it was established as a subspecialty in 2008. Skilled palliative care providers are in growing demand, and the current training capacity has been described as insufficient for ongoing needs (Lupu et al., 2018). Within pediatrics, opportunities for specialty training exist through dedicated hospice and palliative medicine (HPM) fellowships at free-standing children's hospitals or through pediatric tracks within adult HPM fellowships. Some adult fellowships have variable opportunities for some pediatric exposure. Most graduating HPM fellows will not be caring for children. In fact, only 11% of surveyed respondents reported that they would care for pediatric patients more than 50% of their time following fellowship (American Academy of Hospice and Palliative Medicine [AAHPM], 2019a). This highlights the critical importance of high-quality primary pediatric palliative care education.

The momentum for quality palliative care education outreach is currently high. Both the Center to Advance Palliative Care (CAPC) and the National Coalition for Hospice and Palliative Care (NCHPC) have prioritized initiatives to advance PPC through their respective Pediatric Palliative Care National Action Initiative and National Coalition Pediatric Palliative Care Task Force. These initiatives represent national efforts to unite leaders in the palliative care arena to strengthen the field of PPC. Bolstering primary palliative skills for nonpalliative providers has become a priority item for both. For example, CAPC has partnered with the American Academy of Pediatrics and launched a dedicated online skills course for pediatricians on discussing serious illness (AAP, 2020). Similar efforts have had significant impacts. One notable program is the Education in Palliative and End-of-Life Care (EPEC)-Pediatrics program. Funded by a National Institutes of Health and National Cancer Institute R25 grant, a 24-module curriculum delivers online and in-person sessions to teach primary palliative care and offers additional training for graduates so they can become "Master Facilitators," further expanding the outreach of the material (Friedrichsdorf et al., 2019). It has widely been considered the most comprehensive pediatric palliative care education project worldwide (Friedrichsdorf et al., 2019; Postier et al., 2022). With six continents benefiting from this curriculum content, participating clinicians reported perceived improvement in the care of children with serious illness in their regions (Postier et al., 2022). Most children in the world depend on their pediatricians for primary palliative care, and capitalizing on education programs like this is key for comprehensive high-quality pediatric care.

Providers can explore additional avenues for exposure to pediatric palliative care education. These options include institutional or national organizations' continuing medical education (CME) courses, simulation exercises, interdisciplinary certificate programs, and high-quality or sponsored online resources. Many state licensure boards identify and recommend certain CME topics that align with palliative care topics. The most notable include safe opioid prescribing and pain management training (Sinclair & Doodian, 2022). Although not necessarily dedicated to pediatrics, some of these courses offer specific pediatric topics. Importantly, many courses are interdisciplinary, with content applicable to nursing and social work. An important source of educational materials for many pediatric palliative teams and national organizations, such as the American Academy of Pediatrics and American Academy of Hospice and Palliative Medicine, is the Courageous Parents Network. The network is a nonprofit organization that provides resources for families and clinicians based on families' shared experiences dealing with serious illness. Materials readily available to families and clinicians include videos, guided pathways, decision-making guides, and podcasts. This resource has become invaluable for many families and provides clinicians with a wealth of resources to share with patients.

Lastly, graduate and undergraduate medical education across the country has increased palliative care content over the last 40 years (Dickinson, 2011; Fitzpatrick et al., 2017). Additionally, content appears to be more consistent and uniform, which is encouraging (Fitzpatrick et al., 2017). However, medical students and graduating residents are still unprepared when it comes to delivering palliative care (Chen et al., 2015; McCabe et al., 2008; Sullivan et al., 2004). And, unfortunately, it still appears that at the undergraduate level, exposure to consistent pediatric palliative care training is lacking (Fitzpatrick et al., 2017). Furthermore, pediatric residents are graduating from residencies caring for fewer and fewer pediatric patients at the end of life and continue to feel underprepared when entering the workforce (McCabe et al., 2008; Trowbridge et al., 2020). Given limited clinical opportunities to care for children at end of life during residency, palliative simulation exercises have become more important and have demonstrated positive impact on trainee confidence, as discussed in Sect. 5.3.1. Many children's hospitals in the United States do not have a dedicated pediatric hospice and palliative medicine fellowship, let alone fully staffed pediatric palliative care teams (Rogers et al., 2021). Many students and residents interested in pursuing a career in palliative care may experience different educational opportunities depending on region and availability. The AAP's Section on Hospice and Palliative Medicine has worked to provide resources, connect trainees, encourage "away" rotations, provide online platforms for mentorship, and recruit members to national organizations to support the growing need for future pediatric palliative care providers (Humphrey et al., 2023). Medical students and residents alike should seek out dedicated electives at their institutions and look for away rotations, if home institutions are not able to provide the needed exposure. They can additionally depend on a national group of mentors interested in supporting learners, and the AAHPM will offer free membership to students and residents. The hope is that training opportunities will continue to expand and become standard as the field of pediatric palliative care continues to see wide growth.

5.3.1 Simulation and Palliative Care

Palliative care training heavily involves communication skills training. This can be time- and energy-intensive for both the trainees and the educators. Palliative care is a relatively young field in health care, and there continues to be workforce shortages; the need for training opportunities may outmatch the availability of experienced clinicians. Practicing clinicians often develop primary palliative skills over time and with experience. However, especially in pediatrics, trainees are being exposed to fewer deaths, and general comfort with palliative care skills is low (McCabe et al., 2008).

The benefits of simulation in palliative care training have been described in multiple settings and specialties. Skills-based communication training has been developed to train oncology (Back et al., 2003), geriatric (Kelley et al., 2012), and critical care fellows (Arnold et al., 2015). Simulation training has also proven effective in teaching palliative care skills in the general pediatric setting (Taylor et al., 2022), as well as in pediatric fellowships, particularly those in specialties that encounter these high-stakes conversations regularly such as oncology, critical care, cardiology, and neonatology (Brock et al., 2017). Participants reported an increased confidence in talking about death and managing palliative care scenarios (Taylor et al., 2022). It has been used in training of all levels of providers from students through practicing clinicians. It is used in various disciplines, including medicine, nursing, social work, and chaplaincy. Simulation in palliative care training can provide opportunities for learners to practice difficult skills in a setting where they feel safe to attempt new approaches or make mistakes. This can also be a useful method to study and teach provider communication behaviors because researchers can replicate specific scenarios in ways not possible in real patient encounters (Kozhevnikov et al., 2018).

Educators have also used simulation as an opportunity to evaluate trainees' preparedness and skills with conversations (Ross et al., 2017). Skills include providing biomedical information clearly, obtaining the patient's values, talking about uncertainty, giving bad news, conducting a family meeting, helping families reach decisions, negotiating conflict, and recognizing and dealing with one's own feelings. Simulation for palliative care skills has been demonstrated to improve self-reported efficacy in abilities such as relationship building and communicating accurate information, with an improved consultation referral rate to a palliative care team (Brock et al., 2017).

Simulation training is effective in teaching palliative care skills and can be applied to a range of contexts. Given the unpredictable occurrence and nature of "real life" palliative care scenarios, high-quality simulation training in palliative care can augment general and subspecialty pediatric training. This allows learners to increase both confidence and competence in these vital skills and to provide the best possible care during these critical conversations.

5.4 Expanding Equitable Access to Pediatric Palliative Care Nationally and Globally

The need for pediatric hospice and palliative care is growing rapidly, spurred by population growth, increased rates of survival, need for longitudinal support for children with diagnoses such as extreme prematurity and other neurodegenerative diseases, and growing acceptance of both hospice and palliative care. The current US supply of all palliative specialists is 13.35 per 100,000 adults 65 and older (Lupu et al., 2018). While the total number of pediatric palliative physicians in the United States is not well documented, data about the availability of PPC nationally suggests the workforce is inadequate to meet demand. Based on the 2020 National Hospice and Palliative Care Organization (NHPCO) Pediatric Needs Assessment (2023), a large majority of counties do not have access to pediatric palliative services, with 71.5% of counties without access to home-based hospice care, 81.2% without home-based palliative care, 78.7% without inpatient-based hospice care, and 81.5% without inpatient-based palliative care.

A 2020 study evaluated data from 54 PPC programs across the United States that participated in the 2018 National Palliative Care Registry (Rogers et al., 2021). Within these programs, few (37%) met the minimum standards of practice for staffing, with a median of 3.8 full-time equivalent staff per 10,000 hospital admissions (range 0.7–12.1) across the core interdisciplinary team (Rogers et al., 2021). Programs reported being able to provide more annual consults if they were part of long-standing programs at larger hospitals or had more interdisciplinary full-time equivalent staff, which suggests smaller hospitals in underserved areas have less access to PPC. Many programs reported concern for burnout (63%) and an inability to meet clinical demand with available staffing (60%), suggesting that the deficits in access to PPC meet or exceed those of adult palliative care (Rogers et al., 2021).

Access varies across the country by rural and urban settings, and by hospital tax status, with not-for-profit hospitals more likely to provide palliative care. Ninety percent of hospitals with palliative care are in urban areas, and only 17% of rural hospitals with 50 or more beds report palliative care programs (Center to Advance Palliative Care, 2019). Regionally, the south-central United States has the most limited access to palliative care, with less than one-third of hospitals in Arkansas, Mississippi, and Alabama reporting a palliative care team (Center to Advance Palliative Care, 2019).

A 2019 study projected the need for hospice and palliative medicine physicians in 2040 to range from 10,640 to almost 24,000, with supply likely to range from 8100 to 19,000, based on current annual training capacity, which is 325 total new fellows per year (Lupu et al., 2018). As of 2023, there are only 23 pediatric palliative fellowship programs in the United States—two of those being social work fellowships and one being a nurse practitioner fellowship—with a maximum of 32 total slots for pediatric fellows per year (AAHPM, 2023). Given that it is estimated that nearly 180,000 children per year have conditions that warrant palliative care (with this number expected to rise), the deficit for PPC-trained physicians is significant and likely to widen (Institute of Medicine, 2015).

While access to equitable pediatric palliative care remains an ongoing effort in the United States, the need for access to PPC globally surpasses deficits in the United States. Access to PPC worldwide is not well studied, with limited data known about the scale of development of PPC globally, particularly when compared to information about adult palliative care (Clelland et al., 2020). However, a 2016 study suggests that 98% of the global need for PPC comes from low- and middle-income countries (Downing et al., 2016), while the majority of PPC is available in high-income countries. Nearly two-thirds of countries lack access to pediatric palliative care (Knapp et al., 2011), even though children in low- and middle-income countries experience much higher illness-related morbidity and mortality, with strikingly poorer outcomes in terms of cancer survival (Lam et al., 2019). PPC services are considered underdeveloped across Asia, Africa, and Latin America compared to North America and Europe (Zuniga-Villanueva et al., 2021). A 2017 study suggests that 21 million children annually could benefit from some form of palliative care (Connor et al., 2017).

In addition to massive staffing shortages, barriers to access also exist related to provider perceptions of palliative care. In a 2022 survey of 847 Latin American physicians, McNeil et al. (2022) found that while almost all providers expressed a wish to have more training in palliative care, there were gaps in understanding what palliative care means, with 43.4% believing that palliative care equates to end-of-life care. Increasing scholarships and access to PPC training opportunities, including providing virtual options for participation, can also help support capacity building.

Efforts to expand access to PPC fellowship training are part of addressing this need. A novel trilateral partnership between the Unidad Nacional de Oncología Pediátrica in Guatemala City, St. Jude's Children's Research Hospital in Memphis, Tennessee, and the University of Utah in Salt Lake City, Utah, established the first American Council on Graduate Medical Education—International (ACGME-I) pediatric palliative fellowship for Latin American physicians in 2023. This program graduated its first fellow in June 2024, with plans to support two fellows in 2025. The model for this program is informing the development of other ACGME-I PPC fellowship programs, including one in Jordan.

While increasing the number of fellowship-trained PPC physicians is a priority, this alone cannot meet the demand. Various innovative efforts to expand access and capacity have demonstrated positive impact globally. For example, Malawi's Waterloo Coalition Initiative (WCI) provided robust palliative care training over a 10-month period to interdisciplinary health professionals at 13 hospitals in southern Malawi (Kiyange et al., 2024). They then used a cross-sectional evaluation to measure palliative care integration based on 11 consensus-based indicators over a 1-year period and found 92% of participating hospitals made considerable progress in all indicators, including increased pain relief and use of morphine for pediatric patients, where previously no pediatric patients had received morphine for any indication (Kiyange et al., 2024). Community health workers are another underutilized resource that can increase equitable access to palliative care. At Johns Hopkins, the Community Health Worker Intervention for Disparities in Palliative Care (DeCIDE PC) program supports community health workers as care team members to enhance the receipt of palliative care for African Americans with advanced cancer (Siddiqi et al., 2023).

5.4.1 Increasing Underrepresented Identities in Palliative Care

The American Academy of Hospice and Palliative Medicine, which includes a Pediatrics Council comprised of PPC providers across the United States, has formally stated that modeling inclusion and embracing diverse identities of providers and patients is part of improving the quality of palliative care (AAHPM, 2019b). In September 2023, AAHPM began tracking voluntary disclosure of race, ethnicity, sexual orientation, and gender identity of its members to better measure and build a workforce reflecting the diverse patient populations served by hospice and palliative medicine providers.

There remains much work to be done to meet these goals of improved representation. A 2018 survey of all hospice and palliative medicine fellows in the United States ($n = 292$) demonstrated that only 6.8% identified as Hispanic (19.1% of the total US population) and 5.9% as Black (13.6% of the total US population), representing a significant deficit in terms of representation (AAHPM, 2019a). Of these total fellows, only about 11% trained in pediatric specialties that would make them eligible to be board-certified in pediatric settings. Pediatric palliative positions are less available nationally than adult positions, further limiting access to PPC (AAHPM, 2019a).

Pediatric palliative care, like all of medicine, suffers from lack of providers who identify as Black, Hispanic, and Native American, despite the diversity of the patient communities we serve. Given that PPC represents a minority of palliative-trained physicians, and that physicians with marginalized identities are already underrepresented in this group, dedicated efforts to support recruitment, mentorship, and faculty development are vital to correcting this imbalance.

5.4.2 The Role of Palliative Care Providers in Promoting Diversity, Equity, and Inclusion in Our Institutions

Palliative care providers possess a unique skillset that can be leveraged to support diversity, equity, and inclusion efforts at our institutions. Recognizing and responding to instances of abuse and discrimination require an ability to lean into difficult conversations, navigate conflict, and maintain psychological safety, all of which are skills that palliative providers possess (AAHPM, 2019b). Cultivating longitudinal, trusting relationships with families who have experienced marginalization in our health care systems can create space for them to disclose instances of discrimination and receive support and advocacy. At NYU-Langone, the palliative care team has incorporated a universal screening question—"During previous medical encounters have you felt you were treated differently from other patients for any reason?"—that has helped patients trust the medical team and discuss the impacts of racism on their care (Rau et al., 2022).

At our own institution, palliative care providers have been involved in supporting a simulation exercise to help people identify and respond to abuse or mistreatment, based on de-identified cases of witnessed or experienced abuse submitted by our trainees, faculty, and staff. These sessions are informed by palliative communication techniques that involve role-play and debriefing and have shown statistically significant improvement in confidence in responding to microaggressions ($p < 0.01$).

5.5 Conclusion

Pediatric palliative care is a growing field committed to providing holistic, interdisciplinary care for children with life-limiting illness and their families by addressing physical, spiritual, and psychosocial aspects of care. Many specific pediatric populations, from prenatal to adolescents and young adults, face prognostic uncertainty. PPC uniquely supports making significant decisions regarding short- and long-term life-sustaining interventions that align with the goals and values of patients and families. Whether navigating severe neurologic impairment, a cancer relapse, or other life-altering diagnosis, PPC expertise can support complex symptom management, quality of life, shared decision-making, grief, and bereavement. Barriers exist to equitable PPC access by race, ethnicity, language preference, socioeconomic status, insurance coverage, and geographic region. Much work remains to be done to bolster the PPC workforce through increased education and training opportunities, especially for underrepresented providers, and to address systemic barriers to palliative care.

References

American Academy of Hospice and Palliative Medicine (AAHPM). (2019a). *A profile of new hospice and palliative medicine physicians: Results from the survey of hospice and palliative medicine fellows who completed training in 2018.* aahpm.org/uploads/Profile_of_New_HPM_Physicians_2018_June_2019.pdf

American Academy of Hospice and Palliative Medicine (AAHPM). (2019b). *Diversity, equity, and inclusion strategic plan, 2019–2022.* https://aahpm.org/uploads/Final_Revised_D__I_Strategic_Plan_Approved_3_13_19.pdf

American Academy of Hospice and Palliative Medicine (AAHPM). (2023) *Pediatric palliative care fellowships and pediatric tracks.* https://aahpm.org/uploads/Pediatric_Palliative_Care_Fellowships_and_Pediatric_Tracks_Update_06.23.23.pdf

American Academy of Pediatrics (AAP). (2019). Clinical practice guidelines for quality palliative care. *Pediatrics, 143*(1), e20183310. https://doi.org/10.1542/peds.2018-3310

American Academy of Pediatrics (AAP). (2020). *EQIPP: Talking about serious illness.* https://www.aap.org/EQIPP-Talking-About-Serious-Illness

American Academy of Pediatrics (AAP), Committee on Bioethics and Committee on Hospital Care. (2000). Palliative care for children. *Pediatrics, 106*(2), 351–357. https://doi.org/10.1542/peds.106.2.351

American Academy of Pediatrics (AAP), Section on Hospice and Palliative Medicine and Committee on Hospital Care. (2013). Pediatric palliative care and hospice care commitments, guidelines, and recommendations. *Pediatrics, 132*(5), 966–972. https://doi.org/10.1542/peds.2013-2731

Arnold, R. M., Back, A. L., Barnato, A. E., Prendergast, T. J., Emlet, L. L., Karpov, I., White, P. H., & Nelson, J. E. (2015). The critical care communication project: Improving fellows' communication skills. *Journal of Critical Care, 30*(2), 250–254. https://doi.org/10.1016/j.jcrc.2014.11.016

Back, A. L., Arnold, R. M., Tulsky, J. A., Baile, W. F., & Fryer-Edwards, K. A. (2003). Teaching communication skills to medical oncology fellows. *Journal of Clinical Oncology, 21*(12), 2433–2436. https://doi.org/10.1200/JCO.2003.09.073

Beecham, E., Hudson, B. F., Oostendorp, L., Candy, B., Jones, L., Vickerstaff, V., Lakhanpaul, M., Stone, P., Chambers, L., Hall, D., Hall, K., Ganeshamoorthy, T., Comac, M., & Bluebond-Langner, M. (2016). A call for increased paediatric palliative care research: Identifying barriers. *Palliative Medicine, 30*(10), 979–980. https://doi.org/10.1177/0269216316648087

Blume, E. D., Kirsch, R., Cousino, M. K., Walter, J. K., Steiner, J. M., Miller, T. A., Machado, D., Peyton, C., Bacha, E., Morell, E., & American Heart Association Pediatric Heart Failure and Transplantation Committee of the Council on Lifelong Congenital Heart Disease and Heart Health in the Young. (2023). Palliative care across the life span for children with heart disease: A scientific statement from the American Heart Association. *Circulation: Cardiovascular Quality and Outcomes, 16*(2), e000114. https://doi.org/10.1161/HCQ.0000000000000114

Brock, K. E., Cohen, H. J., Sourkes, B. M., Good, J. J., & Halamek, L. P. (2017). Training pediatric fellows in palliative care: A pilot comparison of simulation training and didactic education. *Journal of Palliative Medicine, 20*(10), 1074–1084. https://doi.org/10.1089/jpm.2016.0556

Center to Advance Palliative Care (CAPC). (n.d.) *Clinical training recommendations for all clinicians caring for neonates, perinates, infants, children, adolescents, and/or young adults with serious illness and/or complex needs.* https://www.capc.org/training-recommendations-pediatrics/

Center to Advance Palliative Care, & National Palliative Care Research Center (NPCRC). (2019). *America's care of serious illness.* Retrieved October 18, 2023, from https://reportcard.capc.org/

Chan, A. Y., Ge, M., Harrop, E., Johnson, M., Oulton, K., Skene, S. S., Wong, I. C., Jamieson, L., Howard, R. F., & Liossi, C. (2022). Pain assessment tools in paediatric palliative care: A systematic review of psychometric properties and recommendations for clinical practice. *Palliative Medicine, 36*(1), 30–43.

Chen, E. K., Riffin, C., Reid, M. C., Adelman, R., Warmington, M., Mehta, S. S., & Pillemer, K. (2014). Why is high-quality research on palliative care so hard to do? Barriers to improved research from a survey of palliative care researchers. *Journal of Palliative Medicine, 17*(7), 782–787. https://doi.org/10.1089/jpm.2013.0589

Chen, C. A., Kotliar, D., & Drolet, B. C. (2015). Medical education in the United States: Do residents feel prepared? *Perspectives on Medical Education, 4*(4), 181–185. https://doi.org/10.1007/S40037-015-0194-8

Children's Hospital Association. (n.d.) *Leverage clinical and resource utilization data.* Retrieved January 21, 2024, from https://www.childrenshospitals.org/content/analytics/product-program/pediatric-health-information-system

Clelland, D., van Steijn, D., Macdonald, M. E., Connor, S., Centeno, C., & Clark, D. (2020). Global development of children's palliative care: An international survey of in-nation expert perceptions in 2017. *Wellcome Open Research, 5*, 99. https://doi.org/10.12688/wellcomeopenres.15815.3

Connor, S. R., Downing, J., & Marston, J. (2017). Estimating the global need for palliative care for children: A cross-sectional analysis. *Journal of Pain and Symptom Management, 53*(2), 171–177. https://doi.org/10.1016/j.jpainsymman.2016.08.020

Dickinson, G. E. (2011). Thirty-five years of end-of-life issues in US medical schools. *American Journal of Hospice & Palliative Care, 28*(6), 412–417. https://doi.org/10.1177/1049909110397608

Downing, J., Powell, R. A., Marston, J., Huwa, C., Chandra, L., Garchakova, A., & Harding, R. (2016). Children's palliative care in low- and middle-income countries. *Archives of Disease in Childhood, 101*(1), 85–90. https://doi.org/10.1136/archdischild-2015-308307

Dussel, V., Orellana, L., Holder, R., Porth, R., Avery, M., & Wolfe, J. (2022). A multisite randomized controlled trial of an early palliative care intervention in children with advanced cancer: The PediQUEST Response Study Protocol. *PLoS One, 17*(11), e0277212. https://doi.org/10.1371/journal.pone.0277212

Erçin-Swearinger, H., Lindhorst, T., Curtis, J. R., Starks, H., & Doorenbos, A. Z. (2022). Acute and posttraumatic stress in family members of children with a prolonged stay in a PICU: Secondary analysis of a randomized trial. *Pediatric Critical Care Medicine, 23*(4), 306–314. https://doi.org/10.1097/PCC.0000000000002913

Feudtner, C., Rosenberg, A. R., Boss, R. D., Wiener, L., Lyon, M. E., Hinds, P. S., Bluebond-Langner, M., & Wolfe, J. (2019). Challenges and priorities for pediatric palliative care research in the U.S. and similar practice settings: Report from a Pediatric Palliative Care Research Network workshop. *Journal of Pain and Symptom Management, 58*(5), 909–917.e3. https://doi.org/10.1016/j.jpainsymman.2019.08.011

Fitzpatrick, D., Heah, R., Patten, S., & Ward, H. (2017). Palliative care in undergraduate medical education-how far have we come? *American Journal of Hospice & Palliative Care, 34*(8), 762–773. https://doi.org/10.1177/1049909116659737

Friedel, M., Aujoulat, I., Dubois, A. C., & Degryse, J. M. (2019). Instruments to measure outcomes in pediatric palliative care: A systematic review. *Pediatrics, 143*(1), e20182379. https://doi.org/10.1542/peds.2018-2379

Friedrichsdorf, S. J., Remke, S., Hauser, J., Foster, L., Postier, A., Kolste, A., & Wolfe, J. (2019). Development of a pediatric palliative care curriculum and dissemination model: Education in palliative and end-of-life care (EPEC) pediatrics. *Journal of Pain and Symptom Management, 58*(4), 707–720.e3. https://doi.org/10.1016/j.jpainsymman.2019.06.008

Hasan, F., Widger, K., Sung, L., & Wheaton, L. (2021). End-of-life childhood cancer research: A systematic review. *Pediatrics, 147*(3), e2020003780. https://doi.org/10.1542/peds.2020-003780

Health Measures. (2023). *PROMIS*. Northwestern University. Retrieved February 9, 2024, from https://www.healthmeasures.net/explore-measurement-systems/promis

Humphrey, L., Bhakta, H., Rholl, E. (2023, April). *Pediatric hospice and palliative medicine: A career guide for pediatric residents*. AAP Section on Hospice and Palliative Medicine. Retrieved February 9, 2024, from https://downloads.aap.org/AAP/PDF/2023%20SOHPM%20Career%20Guide%20-%20FINAL.pdf

Institute of Medicine. (2015). Dying in America: Improving quality and honoring individual preferences near the end of life. *Military Medicine, 180*(4), 365–367. https://doi.org/10.7205/MILMED-D-15-00005

Kelley, A. S., Back, A. L., Arnold, R. M., Goldberg, G. R., Lim, B. B., Litrivis, E., Smith, C. B., & O'Neill, L. B. (2012). Geritalk: Communication skills training for geriatric and palliative medicine fellows. *Journal of the American Geriatrics Society, 60*(2), 332–337. https://doi.org/10.1111/j.1532-5415.2011.03787.x

Khoo, E. J., Duenas, D. M., Wilfond, B. S., Gelinas, L., & Antommaria, A. H. M. (2023). Incentives in pediatric research in developing countries: When are they too much? *Pediatrics, 151*(2), e2021055702. https://doi.org/10.1542/peds.2021-055702

Kiyange, F., Atieno, M., Luyirika, E. B. K., Ali, Z., Musau, H., Thambo, L., Rhee, J. Y., Namisango, E., & Rosa, W. E. (2024). Measuring palliative care integration in Malawi through service provision, access, and training indicators: The Waterloo Coalition Initiative. *BMC Palliative Care, 23*(1), 17. https://doi.org/10.1186/s12904-023-01331-0

Knapp, C., Woodworth, L., Wright, M., Downing, J., Drake, R., Fowler-Kerry, S., Hain, R., & Marston, J. (2011). Pediatric palliative care provision around the world: A systematic review. *Pediatric Blood & Cancer, 57*(3), 361–368. https://doi.org/10.1002/pbc.23100

Kozhevnikov, D., Morrison, L. J., & Ellman, M. S. (2018). Simulation training in palliative care: State of the art and future directions. *Advances in Medical Education and Practice, 9*, 915–924. https://doi.org/10.2147/AMEP.S153630

Lam, C. G., Howard, S. C., Bouffet, E., & Pritchard-Jones, K. (2019). Science and health for all children with cancer. *Science, 363*(6432), 1182–1186. https://doi.org/10.1126/science.aaw4892

Lau, N., Bradford, M. C., Steineck, A., Scott, S., Bona, K., Yi-Frazier, J. P., McCauley, E., & Rosenberg, A. R. (2020). Examining key sociodemographic characteristics of adolescents and young adults with cancer: A post hoc analysis of the promoting resilience in stress management randomized clinical trial. *Palliative Medicine, 34*(3), 336–348. https://doi.org/10.1177/0269216319886215

Linebarger, J. S., Collura, C. A., Humphrey, L. M., Miller, E. G., Williams, C. S. P., Rholl, E., Ajayi, T., Lord, B., & McCarty, C. L. (2022). Guidance for pediatric end-of-life care. *Pediatrics, 149*(5), e2022057011. https://doi.org/10.1542/peds.2022-057011

Livingston, J., Cheng, Y. I., Wang, J., Tweddle, M., Friebert, S., Baker, J. N., Thompkins, J., & Lyon, M. E. (2020). Shared spiritual beliefs between adolescents with cancer and their families. *Pediatric Blood & Cancer, 67*(12), e28696. https://doi.org/10.1002/pbc.28696

Lupu, D., Quigley, L., Mehfoud, N., & Salsberg, E. S. (2018). The growing demand for hospice and palliative medicine physicians: Will the supply keep up? *Journal of Pain and Symptom Management, 55*(4), 1216–1223. https://doi.org/10.1016/j.jpainsymman.2018.01.011

Marcus, K. L., Santos, G., Ciapponi, A., Comandé, D., Bilodeau, M., Wolfe, J., & Dussel, V. (2020). Impact of specialized pediatric palliative care: A systematic review. *Journal of Pain and Symptom Management, 59*(2), 339–364. https://doi.org/10.1016/j.jpainsymman.2019.08.005

McCabe, M. E., Hunt, E. A., & Serwint, J. R. (2008). Pediatric residents' clinical and educational experiences with end-of-life care. *Pediatrics, 121*(4), e731–e737. https://doi.org/10.1542/peds.2007-1657

McNeil, M. J., Ehrlich, B. S., Wang, H., Vedaraju, Y., Bustamante, M., Dussel, V., Friedrich, P., Garcia Quintero, X., Gillipelli, S. R., Gomez Garcia, W., Graetz, D. E., Kaye, E. C., Metzger, M. L., Sabato Danon, C. V., Devidas, M., Baker, J. N., & Agulnik, A. (2022). Physician perceptions of palliative care for children with cancer in Latin America. *JAMA Network Open, 5*(3), e221245. https://doi.org/10.1001/jamanetworkopen.2022.1245

Merz, A., Feifer, D., Avery, M., Tsuchiyose, E., Eche, I., Awofeso, O., Wolfe, J., Dussel, V., & Requena, M. L. (2023). Patient-reported outcome benefits for children with advanced cancer and parents: A qualitative study. *Journal of Pain and Symptom Management, 66*(3), e327–e334. https://doi.org/10.1016/j.jpainsymman.2023.05.016

Michelson, K. N., Frader, J., Charleston, E., Rychlik, K., Aniciete, D. Y., Ciolino, J. D., Sorce, L. R., Clayman, M. L., Brown, M., Fragen, P., Malakooti, M., Derrington, S., & White, D. (2020). A randomized comparative trial to evaluate a PICU navigator-based parent support intervention. *Pediatric Critical Care Medicine, 21*(9), e617–e627. https://doi.org/10.1097/PCC.0000000000002378

Mooney-Doyle, K., Pyke-Grimm, K. A., Lanzel, A. F., Montgomery, K. E., Hassan, J., Thompson, A., Rouselle, R., & Antommaria, A. H. M. (2022). Balancing protection and progress in pediatric palliative care research: Stakeholder perspectives. *Pediatrics*, e2022057502. Advance online publication https://doi.org/10.1542/peds.2022-057502

National Consensus Project for Quality Palliative Care. (2018). *Clinical practice guidelines for quality palliative care* (4th ed.). National Coalition for Hospice and Palliative Care. Retrieved October 18, 2023, from https://www.nationalcoalitionhpc.org/ncp

National Hospice and Palliative Care Organization (NHPCO). (2023). *NHPCO pediatric facts and figures* (23rd ed.). National Hospice and Palliative Care Organization. https://www.nhpco.org/wp-content/uploads/NHPCO_Pediatric_Facts_Figures_2023.pdf

Needle, J. S., Friebert, S., Thompkins, J. D., Grossoehme, D. H., Baker, J. N., Jiang, J., Wang, J., & Lyon, M. E. (2022). Effect of the family-centered advance care planning for teens with cancer intervention on sustainability of congruence about end-of-life treatment preferences: A randomized clinical trial. *JAMA Network Open, 5*(7), e2220696. https://doi.org/10.1001/jamanetworkopen.2022.20696

Nelson, K. E., Feinstein, J. A., Gerhardt, C. A., Rosenberg, A. R., Widger, K., Faerber, J. A., & Feudtner, C. (2018). Emerging methodologies in pediatric palliative care research: Six case studies. *Children (Basel), 5*(3), 32. https://doi.org/10.3390/children5030032

Nye, R. T., Hill, D. L., Carroll, K. W., Boyden, J. Y., Katcoff, H., Griffis, H., Campos, D., Hall, M., Wolfe, J., & Feudtner, C. (2022). The design of a data management system for a multi-center palliative care cohort study. *Journal of Pain and Symptom Management, 64*(1), e53–e60. https://doi.org/10.1016/j.jpainsymman.2022.03.006

Papa, S., Mercante, A., Giacomelli, L., & Benini, F. (2023). Pediatric palliative care: Insights into assessment tools and review instruments. *Children (Basel), 10*(8), 1406. https://doi.org/10.3390/children10081406

Pinheiro, L. C., McFatrich, M., Lucas, N., Walker, J. S., Withycombe, J. S., Hinds, P. S., Sung, L., Tomlinson, D., Freyer, D. R., Mack, J. W., Baker, J. N., & Reeve, B. B. (2018). Child and adolescent self-report symptom measurement in pediatric oncology research: A systematic literature review. *Quality of Life Research, 27*(2), 291–319. https://doi.org/10.1007/s11136-017-1692-4

Postier, A. C., Wolfe, J., Hauser, J., Remke, S. S., Baker, J. N., Kolste, A., Dussel, V., Bernadá, M., Widger, K., Rapoport, A., Drake, R., Chong, P. H., & Friedrichsdorf, S. J. (2022). Education in palliative and end-of-life care-pediatrics: Curriculum use and dissemination. *Journal of Pain and Symptom Management, 63*(3), 349–358. https://doi.org/10.1016/j.jpainsymman.2021.11.017

Rau, M., Arora, A., Linton, J., Quest, T., & Milazzo, K. (2022). If you don't ask, you don't get it: Implementation of a discrimination screening question palliative care inpatient consults (ODS5). *Journal of Pain and Symptom Management, 63*(5), 844–845. https://doi.org/10.1016/j.jpainsymman.2022.02.325

Ritchie, C. L., Pollak, K. I., Kehl, K. A., Miller, J. L., & Kutner, J. S. (2017). Better together: The making and maturation of the Palliative Care Research Cooperative Group. *Journal of Palliative Medicine, 20*(6), 584–591. https://doi.org/10.1089/jpm.2017.0138

Rogers, M. M., Friebert, S., Williams, C. S. P., Humphrey, L., Thienprayoon, R., & Klick, J. C. (2021). Pediatric palliative care programs in US hospitals. *Pediatrics, 148*(1), e2020021634. https://doi.org/10.1542/peds.2020-021634

Rosenberg, A. R., Bradford, M. C., Junkins, C. C., Taylor, M., Zhou, C., Sherr, N., Kross, E., Curtis, J. R., & Yi-Frazier, J. P. (2019). Effect of the promoting resilience in stress management intervention for parents of children with cancer (PRISM-P): A randomized clinical trial. *JAMA Network Open, 2*(9), e1911578. https://doi.org/10.1001/jamanetworkopen.2019.11578

Rosenberg, A. R., Zhou, C., Bradford, M. C., Barton, K., Junkins, C. C., Taylor, M., Kross, E. K., Curtis, J. R., Dionne-Odom, J. N., & Yi-Frazier, J. P. (2021). Parent perspectives after the PRISM-P randomized trial: A mixed-methods analysis. *Journal of Palliative Medicine, 24*(10), 1505–1515. https://doi.org/10.1089/jpm.2020.0720

Ross, M. K., Doshi, A., Carrasca, L., Pian, P., Auger, J., Baker, A., Proudfoot, J. A., & Pian, M. S. (2017). Interactive palliative and end-of-life care modules for pediatric residents. *International Journal of Pediatrics, 2017*, 7568091. https://doi.org/10.1155/2017/7568091

Sample, E., Mikulic, C., & Christian-Brandt, A. (2021). Unheard voices: Underrepresented families' perspectives of pediatric palliative care. *Clinical Practice in Pediatric Psychology, 9*(3), 318–322. https://doi.org/10.1037/cpp0000412

Siddiqi, A., Monton, O., Woods, A., Masroor, T., Fuller, S., Owczarzak, J., Yenokyan, G., Cooper, L. A., Freund, K. M., Smith, T. J., Kutner, J. S., Colborn, K. L., Joyner, R., Elk, R., & Johnston, F. M. (2023). Dissemination and implementation of a community health worker intervention for disparities in palliative care (DeCIDE PC): A study protocol for a hybrid type 1 randomized controlled trial. *BMC Palliative Care, 22*(1), 139. https://doi.org/10.1186/s12904-023-01250-0

Sinclair, S., & Doodian, L. (2022, August 23). *Leveraging CME requirements to improve palliative care delivery*. Center to Advance Palliative Care. Retrieved February 13, 2024, from https://www.capc.org/blog/leveraging-cme-requirements-improve-palliative-care-delivery/

Sullivan, A. M., Warren, A. G., Lakoma, M. D., Liaw, K. R., Hwang, D., & Block, S. D. (2004). End-of-life care in the curriculum: A national study of medical education deans. *Academic Medicine, 79*(8), 760–768. https://doi.org/10.1097/00001888-200408000-00011

Taylor, N., Nair, V., & Grimbley, J. (2022). Better general paediatric and neonatal palliative care skills: simulation teaching. *BMJ Supportive & Palliative Care*, bmjspcare-2021-003389. Advance online publication. https://doi.org/10.1136/bmjspcare-2021-003389.

Trowbridge, A., Bamat, T., Griffis, H., McConathey, E., Feudtner, C., & Walter, J. K. (2020). Pediatric resident experience caring for children at the end of life in a children's hospital. *Academic Pediatrics, 20*(1), 81–88. https://doi.org/10.1016/j.acap.2019.07.008

Visser, C., Hadley, G., & Wee, B. (2015). Reality of evidence-based practice in palliative care. *Cancer Biology & Medicine, 12*(3), 193–200. https://doi.org/10.7497/j.issn.2095-3941.2015.0041

Weaver, M. S., Mooney-Doyle, K., Kelly, K. P., Montgomery, K., Newman, A. R., Fortney, C. A., Bell, C. J., Spruit, J. L., Kurtz Uveges, M., Wiener, L., Schmidt, C. M., Madrigal, V. N., & Hinds, P. S. (2019). The benefits and burdens of pediatric palliative care and end-of-life research: A systematic review. *Journal of Palliative Medicine, 22*(8), 915–926. https://doi.org/10.1089/jpm.2018.0483

Wolfe, J., Orellana, L., Cook, E. F., Ullrich, C., Kang, T., Geyer, J. R., Feudtner, C., Weeks, J. C., & Dussel, V. (2014). Improving the care of children with advanced cancer by using an electronic patient-reported feedback intervention: Results from the PediQUEST randomized controlled trial. *Journal of Clinical Oncology, 32*(11), 1119–1126. https://doi.org/10.1200/JCO.2013.51.5981

World Health Organization (WHO). (2018). *Integrating palliative care and symptom relief into paediatrics: A WHO guide for health care planners, implementers and managers.* https://www.who.int/publications/i/item/integrating-palliative-care-and-symptom-relief-into-paediatrics

Zuniga-Villanueva, G., Ramos-Guerrero, J. A., Osio-Saldaña, M., Casas, J. A., Marston, J., & Okhuysen-Cawley, R. (2021). Quality indicators in pediatric palliative care: Considerations for Latin America. *Children (Basel), 8*(3), 250. https://doi.org/10.3390/children8030250

Index